Psychotherapy
for
Mothers and Infants

Psychotherapy
for
Mothers and Infants

Interventions for
Dyads at Risk

Eva R. Grubler Gochman

PRAEGER

Westport, Connecticut
London

Library of Congress Cataloging-in-Publication Data

Gochman, Eva R. Grubler.
    Psychotherapy for mothers and infants : interventions for dyads at
risk / Eva R. Grubler Gochman.
      p. cm.
    Includes bibliographical references and index.
    ISBN 0–275–94927–3 (alk. paper)
    1. Infant psychiatry. 2. Mother and infant. 3. Children of the
mentally ill. 4. Mental illness—Prevention. I. Title.
    [DNLM: 1. Mother–Child Relations. 2. Maternal Behavior—
psychology. 3. Psychotherapy—methods. 4. Mental Disorders—
prevention & control. WS 105.5.F2 G576p 1995]
RJ502.5.G63   1995
618.92′89—dc20
DNLM/DLC
for Library of Congress   94–24215

British Library Cataloguing in Publication Data is available.

Library of Congress Catalog Card Number: 94–24215
ISBN: 0–275–94927–3

First published in 1995

Praeger Publishers, 88 Post Road West, Westport, CT 06881
An imprint of Greenwood Publishing Group, Inc.

Printed in the United States of America

The paper used in this book complies with the
Permanent Paper Standard issued by the National
Information Standards Organization (Z39.48–1984).

10 9 8 7 6 5 4 3 2 1

I dedicate this book, first and foremost, to my children, David and Julie, who have taught me more than anyone about human development and have helped me mature in my mothering. I also dedicate this book to my husband, Stanley, for going down the parenting path together with me, as well as for his intellectual help and support in my work and in the preparation of this book. And I dedicate this book to my parents, David and Josefine Grubler, who struggled with a harsh world to give their children love, security, and joy in learning and exploration.

Finally, I dedicate this book to all the valiant parents who love their children and try to do their best for them to have "a good life."

Contents

Tables

Preface

This book is based on more than three decades of research and clinical psychological work and observation with infants, children, adolescents, and adults in various settings, from hospital to clinic to office, and in various cultures. It brings together the observations and findings of early work at a special school for "atypical" children and faculty appointments at the University of Massachusetts, the University of Maryland, Rutgers University, the University of Puerto Rico, and the American University; clinical work and research at Topeka State Hospital in association with the Menninger Foundation, work at the Veterans Administration, the Somerset County (New Jersey) Guidance Center, the Bergen Center for Psychological Services and the Institute for Analytic Psychotherapy (New Jersey), the Peace Corps (for Latin America), and St. Elizabeths Hospital/ the National Institute for Mental Health (NIMH), and with the District of Columbia Commission on Mental Health Services; and, for the latter two, ten years directing the Parent and Infant Development Program.

It brings together findings from both public and private practice, from work with ethnic groups—Hispanics, African Americans, and others— with the spectrum of upper and lower socioeconomic groups, including those truly at the bottom, the homeless and the "underclass," and across the continuum of human behavior from those relatively normal to those floridly psychotic.

Remarkably, focused psychotherapy for the prevention of psychopathology in at-risk children does work. The author would like to share the concepts and methods of this psychotherapy with the reader.

For the first time, focused preventive intervention is applied to worst case scenarios—the psychotic hospitalized and the severely disturbed, schizophrenia, bipolar, major depression, and substance abuse—for the prevention of psychopathology in their children.

One would like to think that the program has already had some impact upon mental health services in the national capital area and, through presentations and seminars, at a national level. Since it began at one of the centers of NIMH resources, it has perhaps ignited the beginnings of a carry-over to the development of training and research in primary prevention programs within NIMH. The author hopes that it has stimulated, and will continue to stimulate, others to begin clinical and research work in this area in both the public and the private sector.

This report begins with the case of "Mary" and goes on to discuss the body of research, theory, and practice that has grown up around working with infants, parents, and parents-to-be. I have named this type of clinical intervention parent-infant *dyadic psychotherapy*.

Introduction

It has been generally acknowledged, within recent years, that the early experiences of the child impact his/her later development. That is, the child's (e.g., Greenspan, 1987; Werner, 1989) and then the adult's level of emotional and total functioning has its foundations in the earliest years. Perhaps equally important, the quality and vector of the relationship between parent(s) and child develop their grounding and direction during the earliest years of interaction and attachment formation. The importance of the parent(s)' specific interactions and emotional harmony with the child has become increasingly highlighted.

However, together with this heightened understanding, societal changes have been taking place that go counter to the needs of the developing child. The "family" has changed profoundly. Single parent families proliferate, contracting out of child care increases, and societal complexities and stresses increase.

Infants are the most needy of continuous, consistent, emotionally attuned caretaking, and are at the same time the most helpless to demand this and to effect fulfillment of their needs. Infants are also the future children, adolescents, and adults of society—in fact, our very future.

We have already seen effects of the breakdown of the family in the increase in counter-societal trends. We need emotionally and psychologically well-developed people if we want society to develop in a positive direction, which will serve the needs of its constituents.

I write this book in the hope that it will promote the well-being of individuals directly benefiting from psychotherapeutic interventions, as well as the well-being of society collectively, which depends on the sum of its parts.

1

The Case of Mary

The "Case of Mary" introduces the reader to a worst case scenario, the case of a young mother-to-be. This is a multi-risk situation: the woman is a poor, inner-city, black woman who has been both homeless and hospitalized for major mental illness.

How does one begin to work with such an at-risk mother-to-be? How does Mary react? How does Mary treat her infant? How does Mary's psychopathology and disordered thinking affect her child care and her infant's development? How does the therapist intervene in order to help Mary, change her thinking, and modify her behavior? How does the therapist work on the primary prevention of psychopathology in Mary's infant? What is the beginning therapist to look for and to do? What are the implications and conclusions from Mary's case that apply and transfer to the "average" American mother? These are some of the issues that the "Case of Mary" begins to develop and that will be explored in later chapters.

Mary was a pretty young woman, but one wouldn't know it. She was sitting still, looking down. She was visibly pregnant. When her therapist introduced herself, Mary hardly reacted. She was having a baby in a few weeks. How would this impassive woman take care of her child? How did she get like this? Could she be helped?

Mary had grown up in a household that did not welcome her birth and did not concern itself with her day-to-day well-being and little hurts. Her mother was well known to the mental health center. Her father had left the family long ago. Some of her aunts and uncles had been patients in a mental hospital and/or had been incarcerated. Mary was a defiant teenager. She felt unloved. Her mother's boyfriend made sexual advances toward her. She started to act out with the boys in the neighborhood. When she became a teenager, she also became pregnant. Unable to care for the baby, a relative was found who would bring him up. Mary's mother was furious about her condition. Mary had a second child whom another relative took. The fights at home were terrible and terrifying. Her mother threw her out of the house; then a period of homelessness followed. It was terrible not to know where she would be sleeping. She met Tom at this time. They were homeless together for three years; now she was so depressed that she had been admitted to the hospital.

Her therapist talked to her, asked her to tell her about herself, how she felt, what she was looking forward to, her plans. Mary said little. She had learned not to trust people. She was confused. She was looking forward to having her baby, but she was afraid of the future. She wanted to keep the baby. She wanted a place of her own. She wanted Tom to live with her. She wanted furniture. She wanted enough money. She wanted a normal life. She sat slumped, perfectly still, looking down. Her voice was barely audible. She looked unkempt and untidy.

It was decided that she would be seen once a week for an hour of pregnancy-oriented psychotherapy. She readily agreed. She knew she was in need of something, but didn't know exactly what. There was a terrible feeling of emptiness.

Mary came to her appointments faithfully. She continued in her unresponsive manner for several sessions. Gradually she became a bit more talkative. She talked about herself, her fears, her hopelessness. She talked about Tom and his loyalty to her, but also about his anger and explosiveness. She talked about her early years of fear, about the harshness of her mother, her feelings hurt by her mother's preference for the other children, her "ugly duckling" feelings. She talked about her hallucinations, the voices she heard. She talked about her timidity and her anger. She talked about the death of a beloved uncle when she was a girl, and her experience that he signaled her from his coffin. She talked about not having a place for her baby-to-be. She talked shyly and indistinctly.

Slowly, over many weeks, her speech became a little clearer, easier to understand. The predominant emotion was her underlying fear. She was afraid she was no good, that she was ugly, that she was not capable of taking care of the baby. She was afraid of her mother, of all people, of losing the baby.

She did not have the psychic energy needed to live her life in an effective manner, to capture the moment, to enjoy the pleasant, to apply reason to problems, or to plan her life. She lived suspended in a timeless world, hoping to survive by being non-animated and by impacting on others as little as possible. But time passed, and Mary had her baby.

She brought her baby to the therapist for the first visit dressed cozily and wrapped in a receiving blanket. Her face was blank. She sat down on the couch, baby across her lap, waiting for the therapist. The therapist's fuss over how cute the baby was caused her to look down for the first time at the baby. Through the therapist's eyes she saw her baby as cute, as responsive, and as gratifying to her. She started to admire the baby and so to feel herself a mother, to feel that this was her baby and that she was "something" to have had a baby.

Mary and her baby had not been welcomed and admired on coming home from the hospital. Mary's mother had not said "welcome home" to her and had not said "what a wonderful baby!" Instead, Mary was merely allowed into the house and tolerated there. She tried hard to take care of her baby. She was very lonely. Though there were others in the house, she was ignored and alone. She always felt that she had to be careful to do things right and not offend the others or get in their way. She was afraid that otherwise she would be thrown out of the house.

Her mother also started to inflict her own child-raising ideas on Mary. These were sometimes contrary to what Mary was told by her pediatrician and sometimes contained rituals to "protect" the baby. Mary felt she had to conform to her mother's wishes. Sometimes Mary's mother accused her of stealing Mary's own food or money. Mary was haunted by feelings of guilt in these accusations, even though she knew she was clearly innocent of any wrongdoing. Her feelings of guilt were so ingrained that little was needed to make them surface. Her preoccupations kept her from interacting with her baby and obtaining joy from her. Her natural interaction was minimal and rigid.

The way in which she held her baby was stiff and unaccommodating. She tended not to look at the baby and avoided eye contact with her. She was quiet, not talking to the baby, nor making sounds or singing to her. She typically put her baby across her lap, without holding her. There was very little movement of the baby. Though there was a rocking chair in the room, this remained unused. Mary's natural mode was to sit quietly, rigidly, with her baby lying across her lap.

The therapist, knowing that infants require stimulation, contingent interaction, and a sense of security in order to thrive, worked with the mother and infant to achieve these. However, the therapist realized that telling Mary how to handle her baby would threaten both her insecure sense of motherhood and also her therapeutic alliance with the therapist.

She therefore tried not to use this means of intervention. She tried to intervene through supportive means in order to encourage the mother to nurture her infant on her own. The therapist also verbalized Mary's own inner reactions to her baby for her. She also verbalized the infant's reactions for Mary. Phrases such as "the baby likes it when you look in her eyes," "the baby feels good when you hold her close and she likes it when you talk to her," "you really feel good when your baby looks in your eyes" abounded.

These verbalizations helped Mary realize she had feelings in relation to the child and helped her clarify them. They also helped her notice the baby's reactions to her and to enjoy them. They elicited the first signs of an awareness of her own sense of pleasure. Since Mary could now begin to take some joy from her interactions with the baby, and since she was able to realize that she had an impact upon her, an interactive cycle of play between mother and infant was set in motion.

Of course there was a good deal of fear on Mary's part. Since Mary felt she herself was bad, she was afraid of her own impulses in relation to the child. This needed to be dealt with psychotherapeutically. Her own sense of lack of control in relation to these impulses that were driving her in a psychotic maelstrom was highly disruptive. A psychotic "core," issue to be discussed later, was collided with in passing by the therapist and interpreted immediately, so that it never had to darken Mary's door again. Her fear came up and was dealt with psychotherapeutically. The therapist's interventions prevented the development of a punitive and fearful interaction cycle between mother and child.

Mary's projections of her own fears and impulses onto the baby also showed themselves. For example, her fear of her own "craziness" was projected onto the baby. She said "her eyes are rolling up." In the context of the tendency for her own eyes to roll up due to medication, and also having seen this phenomenon in other patients on certain psychotropic medication, this became a projection of her own state onto the baby, as well as her prophecy of the future. An immediate preventive intervention here by the therapist forestalled the development of this thought into a fixed idea.

With the therapist's support, the allaying of some of her anxieties about mothering, and her increasing gratification in her interactions with the baby, Mary started to feel good about herself as a mother. She started to have more confidence in how she cared for her baby, and indeed was more attentive, concerned, and interactive with her. She took joy in the baby. She noticed her increasing competencies and was proud. She was pleased with others' reactions to her. Despite her continued personal conflicts and difficulties, she was able to keep these separate from the baby. She was able to interact nurturingly with good feelings about herself and her baby.

The baby in turn, though quite small at birth, thrived. She developed well, reaching the developmental milestones within the normal age limits. She was emotionally responsive and predominantly happy. She was curious, investigating her environment appropriately. Her attention span was good and she learned well. She was not distracted by her own anxieties nor the need to perform for attention. People's spontaneous reactions to her were uniformly positive and typically friendly.

Though Mary had had two previous children, she had not had the experience of motherhood with either of them. She now felt herself a mother. She was highly gratified by this, and it sustained her through subsequent travails. She did not have another pregnancy, since she felt she had accomplished the true sense of motherhood with this child. (Typically, I find there are repeated pregnancies in an effort by poorly attached mothers to feel fulfilled.) She also felt somewhat more at peace with herself, though many problems remained. She continued to have both intrapsychic problems and problems with her environment. However, she was able to maintain herself essentially as an out-patient in the mental health system, whereas previously she had been a revolving-door patient for years. Mary benefited greatly from her three years of *dyadic psychotherapy*. Baby was developing on target.

SOME QUESTIONS AND ANSWERS

Why was Mary looking down and hardly reacting when she first met her therapist?

Mary had lost her ability to react to other people. She had no energy to allow herself to feel emotions or to hope for anything for herself. She had had previous children, but she had not been the caretaker of any of them. They had been removed from her at birth or very soon thereafter.

Mary typically tended to avoid eye contact. She did so in the therapy situation. Eye contact is a major modality for relatedness to other people. Since Mary did not have a feeling of relatedness to other people, she tended to avoid eye contact with them. Lack of eye contact may also have more specific psychodynamics: it may denote shyness, a fear of hurting the other person, or fear of being hurt by the other, in a concretization of internal impulses and projections. However, the predominant reason for her lack of eye contact was that eye contact is the main channel for the development of relatedness to other people. Mary was too afraid because she felt she could not relate to other people, including the therapist. Her expectations were always of rejection and she therefore expected the therapist to reject her as well. However, she came to the therapy situation and sat there conflicted, hoping for acceptance, relatedness with the therapist, and help from her but not expecting it. She was also hoping to develop a relatedness with her baby, but did not expect it.

How would an impassive woman like this take care of her new child?
It is clear that she would not be able to sustain a nurturing relationship to her child in her present state. Mary's lack of eye contact with other people meant that she would tend to do the same with her baby since, as previously stated, eye contact is the main channel for developing an emotional relationship with another person. The lack of eye contact would interfere with the development of the relationship between mother and child. In other words, the attachment process would be interfered with by this lack. A general lack of reactivity also includes a tendency not to talk or to respond in other ways to other people, which would transfer to the child. Mary would tend not to make sounds, talk, or interact verbally with her new baby. This would limit the amount of auditory stimulation for the child and consequently later limit the development of language. If Mary were consistent in her lack of auditory stimulation over time, which is the probability, she would not provide enough language stimulation for the baby to develop language at an adequate level.

Furthermore, Mary's rigidity or lack of reactivity in terms of her own body movements also foretold a probable lack of holding and molding in relation to the baby, which is a natural mothering behavior and is necessary for the baby's development of a sense of security and emotional warmth. This lack of movement on the mother's part would also interfere with the child's emotional development. It could also be anticipated that she would tend not to move the baby, in the sense of rocking or playing with her. Consequently the vestibular sensory mechanism, which is an important element in the development of the total sensorium of the baby, would also tend not to be stimulated. In most instances, where there is no substantial interference due to psychopathology, this interaction between mother and baby occurs naturally.

What has not been mentioned so far is the ability of the mother to deal conceptually with the child—her ability to make decisions as to when the child should sleep or about when and how to feed the baby. Any decisions by the mother would of course be influenced by her emotions as well. Even if she were able to make rational decisions concerning the amount of food and the timing of feeding and sleeping—decisions regarding the biological necessities of the child—there would still be problems in the way she went about it. From the very beginning of interaction between mother and child a pattern of interaction is set up. The mother who does not make eye contact with her baby does not allow the baby to make eye contact with her, and so the baby does not have the opportunity to develop a feeling of closeness and interaction with the mother. Consequently the baby, in not feeling a closeness or relatedness to the mother, will stop trying to establish the relatedness. The mother, in turn, will react to the baby's not seeking eye contact, for example, as rejection, which will confirm her hypothesis that people reject her, including her own baby. This would tend to reinforce all of the feelings she has about others and how they react to her. This would then tend to complete the cycle of her distancing herself even more from the baby. Feelings of anger may then also surface in her feelings toward the baby. These would manifest themselves in her interaction with the child, so that minimally the tension of her muscles as she holds the baby would be affected. Her affect, in her total interactions with the baby, would then tend to become one of anger. Since the baby has very strong biological needs that require the caretaker to act to meet them, when they are not met the baby will cry. That cry is probably the most compelling and irritating sound imaginable when it escalates. The mother who has not attached to that child adequately will only be irritated by it and again will tend to react with anger. Consequently a vicious cycle is started in the interaction process between mother and child. Unless something changes within the mother, within the child, or in the circumstances, or another person is introduced into the situation, this pattern tends to remain, cement itself, and increase in intensity. We would then have the foundations of an abrasive, hostile relationship between parent and child.

Why is it that after Mary had her first child, as a teenager, and the child was taken by a relative, that she got pregnant again and had another child?

Women who have felt all alone in the world on an emotional level, who have felt rejected and unwanted, nevertheless continue to hope for a relationship with another human being. They continue to hope for acceptance and love. Typically, if there is a pregnancy, this woman will tend to hope for all of these things to be forthcoming from the baby, often on an unconscious level. In other words, she will hope that her needs will be met by this new person who belongs to her. The feeling that "this is my baby, a product of myself," gives the mother the feeling and the hope that this part of herself will love her. Consequently, in the pregnancy, even though it may be an "unwanted" pregnancy, there is always an ambivalence between wanting and not wanting the child. The child is wanted for the mother's emotional fulfillment and also frequently to fulfill social needs in relation to friends and family, whom the pregnant woman hopes will look upon her differently, in a more respectful or serious way. She hopes to be regarded as a real person because she has had a baby. Teenagers are typically considered, or are in fact, unable to take care of their own baby. Consequently, as in this case, the child was removed. The emotional needs of the mother, however, remained. Therefore, the tendency is that if the baby is removed from the mother, she will soon get pregnant again to try to replace that child, with the same emotions and hopes that she had initially. For example, in this case Mary had her second pregnancy soon after the first, though she knew that her mother would be very angry, in fact furious, about the second pregnancy. The need to have someone who would accept her, in the form of the baby, was greater. There is the additional trauma of loss when the baby is removed—the loss of an object that had the potential to supply love to the mother.

Why did Mary's speech become clearer and easier to understand after some weeks of therapy?

Mary was in a state of limited reactivity when she started therapy. This included her reactivity in speech. She did not think clearly and verbalized little. When she did verbalize, she was not able to do so clearly or well. Her state was not the same as, but somewhat akin to, that of someone just falling asleep, or just waking up, when there is not a full, clear sensorium or ability to think. Also, depression was present, which had lifted to some extent. Depression would tend to suppress the productivity in language. The clarity of her speech was affected by a lack of practice. She generally spoke little. Her speech production was as though she were enmeshed in clouds or cotton, making it hard for her to think or speak clearly. After having had the opportunity to vent some of her feelings, some of her depression lifted. She was able to develop a sense that there was someone who was interested in her. More important, she began to feel that there must be something about her that made it possible for another person to be interested in her. She developed a sense of some relatedness to the world and to others, a sense of being. This allowed her to have enough awareness and assertiveness to speak in such a way as to be able to be understood.

Why is it so very important to be "welcomed home" and admired with a new baby?

It is natural to want and seek admiration for any new acquisition, even for a pair of new shoes. We tend to take delight in the admiration that others show for our choices, our possessions, or anything new that we acquire.

In a normal family situation, the most natural reaction is that when a mother has a new baby, the immediate and the extended family, friends and neighbors, will admire the new baby. The mother basks in the admiration of her product. Since the baby is not merely an acquired object but a product most directly of herself, it is a very powerful and meaningful event when a mother receives admiration for her baby. The mother's experience is that this admiration is for her as well, that it is part of herself that is being admired. This expression of admiration tends to reinforce very strongly the mother's own perception of her baby. This process is typically not even noticed because it is such an integral part of the fabric of our lives. It may not even be noted as a phenomenon. However, when this admiration is missing, it is critical. We see this in the case of Mary, who received no admiration or even comment concerning her baby from her family. Mary, already emotionally blunted, was additionally deprived of this stimulus for herself in developing a relatedness to the baby. The therapist, in providing this admiration, provided a very powerful stimulus and support to the mother, who so keenly needed it.

Why did Mary feel that she had to conform to her mother's wishes on baby care?

Passing along ideas of baby care from one generation to the next is, generally speaking, a helpful means of maintaining the culture in which we find ourselves. However, problems arise when there is an imposition of dictums on baby care, which the mother feels are not in the interests of her child, and to which she does not want to conform, and yet from which she cannot free herself or is not strong enough to resist. Mary's mother imposed dictums upon her which included ritualistic procedures that Mary did not want to carry out. Nevertheless she had a compulsion to conform to her mother's wishes. Mary had so little ego strength at this time that she sought her own dependence on her mother. She was perhaps even grateful for the attention received from her mother, even though she felt it was negative. She wanted so much to be accepted by her mother that she had great difficulty in resisting her suggestions on the care of her baby. Some degree of magical thinking can also be involved, as in this case, where a fear is present that if she does not conform, something bad will happen to the child or perhaps to her. A conflict develops between her following these dictums and not doing so. The conflict consumes much of her energy and consequently interferes with her spontaneous and more joyful interactions with the baby. She is very preoccupied with doing the right thing and is consumed by the conflict between doing what her mother wants her to do or what she feels is correct.

What is the importance of stimulation for the baby?

In fact, all people need stimulation throughout their life span. When stimulation is lacking, the functions that are not stimulated tend to diminish. For the baby, stimulation is critically important. We do not typically notice this because in the normal family situation the baby receives the necessary stimulation. There is stroking and playing with the baby. People come and pick him/her up. There is touching, eye contact, rocking, movement, and cuddling. These are all things that the baby needs. It is only when such stimulation is lacking that we notice its effect. For instance, babies who are not picked up sufficiently, who do not receive the stimulation of being moved around, try to make up for that by stimulating themselves. Some do this by rocking themselves when they get old enough to do so. In extreme cases, a child will rock incessantly.

Children who do not hear speech, do not develop speech. It is again necessary to have the stimulation to enable that sensory area to develop and for learning to take place. At the extreme, there are structural changes that take place with lack of stimulation. The baby's eyes require the stimulation of patterns of light, otherwise structural changes occur that will eventually make it difficult for vision to develop. This is particularly true during infancy. The same principle is true in each area of functioning. Stimulation is necessary in each area for the functions to develop adequately.

Stimulation of a gentle, nurturing manner is intrinsic in interaction of mother and child, leading to attachment between them. The quality of this attachment then forms the basis for the quality of continuing reciprocal interactions and relationship.

What is the importance of contingent mother-infant interactions?

When the baby cries, the mother will come and see what to do about that. For instance, if she finds that the baby is hungry, she will feed the baby. The baby learns that it will get a response from the mother if it communicates its needs to her. The mother will feed the baby contingent on its demand for food. She will respond to the baby's eye contact by looking in its eyes. When the baby babbles, she will talk baby talk. This contingent type of interaction helps the development of the relationship between mother and baby. And, most important, it helps the baby develop the feeling that it is capable of having an impact on the mother. In other words, the feeling that it has some degree of power. When contingent reactions are consistently not forthcoming from the mother, the baby will learn that. After some learning of non-contingency in feeding, for example, the baby may cease to cry for food. If the baby has learned non-contingency in eye contact, the baby may cease to try to catch the mother's eye. The contingent reaction of the mother is important in the baby's development of a sense of self and of a sense of power in participating in the process of getting its needs met.

How is it that if the therapist were to tell Mary how to handle her baby, this would threaten the therapeutic alliance she had established with the therapist?

The patient develops a relationship with the therapist, which is called a therapeutic alliance, on the basis of developing a sense of support from the therapist, as well as the feeling that the therapist is working with her to help her feel more comfortable with herself. In dyadic psychotherapy, additionally, the patient feels that the therapist is there to help her in her relationship with her baby. If the therapist were to present herself as the expert on child care, this would be in contradiction to the relationship that has been established, the therapeutic alliance. Through the therapeutic alliance the patient has learned to feel increasingly more confirmed in the validity of her own reactions and feelings. What has enabled her to accomplish this is the atmosphere of support and understanding in the therapy.

Within the therapy, the mother's positive behaviors toward the baby have been reinforced. She has been able to develop a sense of freedom, has been able to expand her repertoire of reactions, and to increase her awareness of her own feelings toward the baby. In contrast, she had previously been used to being treated judgmentally and always having to be on the defensive, on the lookout for criticism. She had been given the feeling that she was generally incapable and not a good person. The therapist's giving explicit directions on how she should handle her baby is typically counterindicated in order to safeguard the therapeutic alliance, as well as the mother's good progress of expanding her repertoire of experienced emotions and reactions.

Why is it that Mary herself felt that she was bad and that she was afraid of her own impulses in relation to the child?

The feeling of being a bad person typically comes from having experienced a great deal of criticism and implicit rejection, if not overt rejection, in the family during the early years of childhood. The child tends to attribute the cause of rejection and criticism to itself. The attribution typically follows this pattern: "there must be a reason why I'm being treated this way"; the basic experienced reason always comes down to a sense of being bad. This creates a good deal of fear and anger. The anger is easily translated into hostile impulses, which are experienced in relation to other people. The mother's own child is another person, with whom there is a great deal of contact. Furthermore, the child is helpless to defend itself effectively or to retaliate. Consequently, the child makes a good target for hostile feelings and aggression and becomes an easily used object for purposes of venting aggression. It is indeed appropriate for people like Mary to be afraid of their own impulses in relation to their children, to try to control these, and to try to get help to diminish them. These aggressive and hostile impulses are typically extremely disturbing, particularly if they have a strong pressure behind them. They tend to be disruptive of the person's functioning and control systems.

How is it that Mary projected her own fears onto her new baby when she said her eyes were rolling up?

It is a fairly common defense mechanism for people to project their own fears and emotions onto others. Parents tend to experience the child as an extended part of themselves. They readily tend to project their own ego-alien characteristics, feelings, and impulses onto their own children. It is not an infrequent phenomenon that parents are angry at their children for the very characteristics that are really the parents' own. In the case of Mary, she was projecting her own feelings of craziness and inadequacy onto the baby. The way in which she let the therapist know this was by making the statement that she baby was rolling her eyes up. The patient's allowing her unconscious material to surface in her verbalizations is like an escape valve. It is done cautiously, so that if the sensitivity of the therapist should not be available at that moment, that cue will be missed. The patient thereby protects herself. If the therapist does not pick up on the cue, she will not be hurt by her own unconscious coming into awareness without the support of the therapist. If the therapist does pick up on the verbalization, then the therapist is being sensitive at that moment. The patient is therefore encouraged that the therapist will tend to treat the issue sensitively.

How is the baby able to reach the developmental milestones within the normal age ranges?

Mary avoided some of the negative, punitive manners of interacting with her baby which would have developed without the therapy. She did not exhibit high levels of anxiety in relation to the baby. Furthermore, she was sufficiently reactive and stimulating to her. The amount and quality of the interaction were at least good enough to allow the child to develop adequately.

What is the importance of other people's spontaneously reacting to Mary's baby positively and in a friendly way?

The baby's spontaneity and happiness were elicited as others—acquaintances, family members, other professionals, and so on—came in contact with her. The result of Mary's adequate nurturing of her baby resulted in the development of an emotionally competent baby. This, in turn, stimulated other people to react positively, in a pleasant manner and with smiles, to this baby, which in turn further reinforced postive affective reactions. This again stimulated the mother to continue to react positively to the baby.

How is it that Mary had problems in her life despite this dyadic therapeutic intervention?

Mary continued to live in a toxic environment, in both the family and social domains. She continued to live with her toxic mother and in a neighborhood that is considered dangerous. Her friends, including the father of this baby, did not change substantially. The baby's father continued to be a problem to her, having his own substantial psychopathology. She was now able to deal more effectively with all these issues and circumstances but was still enmeshed in them. The therapeutic interventions did help her to deal with them more effectively. She now experienced herself as a real mother. She felt herself the psychological mother of this child. In general, being a good mother is an extremely important aspect of women's lives. The feeling that one has accomplished this is of the highest importance. It helped Mary to have a much better image of herself. Her improved self-concept bolstered her total sense of well-being.

2

Some General Considerations about Pregnancy-Oriented Psychotherapy

This chapter introduces some general considerations that lie along the continuum of infant-focused psychotherapy, from a pregnancy-oriented psychotherapy to a later parent-infant dyadic psychotherapy.

Pregnancy, which is experienced by the average woman as a major life change, is perceived as a major crisis by the emotionally disturbed woman. Yet pregnancy offers the client a special opportunity for change, during the period of pregnancy itself and shortly thereafter. There is a kind of utilizable motivation stimulated by this profound life event that is deep and powerful.

Psychotherapy, particularly for at-risk cases, is best when started during pregnancy. The overriding goal of psychological interventions is to enable the infant to have an adequate developmental base from the earliest time possible.

Specific interventions stem from concepts derived from the broad field of dynamic psychotherapy and psychoanalysis. These concepts, however, are applied and focused on areas of concern related to the special time and condition of pregnancy. Issues dealing with fears, self-concept, perception of oneself as a mother-to-be, and attitudes related to the baby-to-be are explored. A woman's/parent's resultant enhanced ability to deal with these issues more realistically, and to come to terms with her own reality, helps her bring a new baby into the world more effectively.

This chapter discusses some of the most important general prenatal issues in pregnancy-oriented psychotherapy. It begins with those most in need of help, the most severely disturbed and even psychotic parents-to-be. Human behavior exists in a continuum, therefore lessons can be drawn from this group at the extreme of the spectrum which can reasonably apply to the social norm, the average parent-to-be in our society.

PREGNANCY IN THE EMOTIONALLY DISTURBED

Pregnancy, for all women, is physically, psychologically, and socially a major change point in life. The emotionally disturbed woman, however, may well experience pregnancy as a major life crisis. The bodily changes in pregnancy are one general source of intrapsychic stress. The most severely disturbed women may tend to deny the pregnancy per se, or the bodily changes, remaining apparently oblivious to them. Severe depression, when present, may also have the effect of the woman seemingly being nearly unaware of the changes. Changes in shape and body image may create conflicts in the narcissistic personality. There may be resentment toward the father and/or the baby-to-be for these changes in appearance. Changes in appetite may harbor problems in adjustment and may give the woman in need of nurturance an excuse for self-indulgence in eating habits. The more seriously disturbed person is prone to have ideation related to fears of harming the fetus. These thoughts may at first appear to be rational but in fact may be exaggerated concerns. For example, one mother had a great deal of anxiety about her smoking, fearing that it would harm the fetus. This was based on reality, yet her degree of preoccupation with her smoking and inability to control it indicated a tendency toward the delusional. A more extreme psychotic example would be a mother-to-be with a fear of being eaten away by the fetus. Such fears raise the general anxiety level of the patient and interfere with her readiness for parturition and motherhood.

Another general source of stress is the knowledge that a new baby will be making its entrance into the world. All of the related issues may become sources of stress. For example, the relationship with the baby's father may be predominantly positive or negative. He may be happy about the pregnancy or may not. He may be rejecting, hostile, and/or aggressive. He may or may not accept some responsibility for the child. Since interpersonal relationships for women with severe emotional problems are typically tenuous, these have often been severed either prior to or soon after the birth of a baby. Conflicts and hurts surround these insecure relationships. Being alone or feeling alone is particularly painful at this time, when all women feel, and are, at their most vulnerable, in their need to be cared for. Frequently, the emotionally disturbed mother has over the years alienated her family of origin, and so they will not help her further. The family of origin itself typically has long-standing, dysfunctional emotional problems. This leaves the severely emotionally disturbed mother-to-be without family support, a difficult condition for anyone, but in this case devastating. Even when there are family members in the household, the mother-to-be tends to feel alineated and lonely. For instance, one mother-to-be lived with her own mother, as well as with her sister and her sister's family. She slept in the living room and was very quiet and non-demanding, because she felt constantly fearful that her family would throw her out of the house.

Basic questions as to housing, food, and resources available to care for the physical well-being of the infant may raise anxieties. Many emotionally debilitated women deny these anxieties and thereby the problem, and do not try to plan ahead. The very idea that one should *not* plan ahead is not unusual in pregnant women: there is magical thinking involved with fears for the baby or oneself. The myth that planning for the baby-to-be will harm the child is fairly widespread. The degree to which the myth is adhered to varies greatly. When it totally interferes with planning, it becomes a serious detriment for the isolated mother who is then ill-equipped for the care of the new infant. When these fears are deep-seated in the psyche, they cannot easily be dispelled through educational means.

Psychotherapeutic intervention, on the other hand, can be of great help. Conflicts as to whether to maintain the pregnancy, or whether to keep the child, for example, may be unresolved. These conflicts may be quite powerful. The woman may, for instance, not want to have a baby, but feel that she is bad for having such feelings. Having a baby, or not having a baby, may be a form of acting out for the woman. For example, one woman said she would get an abortion, until a helpful relative suggested she do so. She then stated that she would have the baby, in order to spite her relative. The last thing she would do was take her relative's advice.

Childbirth itself is very often perceived as a crisis even by the average woman. There tends to be fear and anxiety associated with parturition, and these increase the difficulty of the childbearing process. Furthermore, there is typically the normal experience of overwhelming pain in labor. Because of the inescapable intensity of the pain, the woman in labor often needs to find an explanation for it. As children, people have been taught that if they are bad, or do something bad, they will be punished. Therefore, when the adult experiences acute pain, the tendency is to interpret this as punishment: "What did I do to deserve this?" In other words, there is backward reasoning: "I am in pain because I am bad." A woman who does not basically see herself as bad will be able to overcome this normal reaction. However, a severely disturbed woman, who generally sees herself as bad and has chronic hostile-aggressive impulses and deep-seated guilt feelings, will have difficulty with the experience of pain. In the extreme, she may develop a psychotic reaction such as postpartum psychosis. It is, of course, terribly unfortunate should this largely preventable condition be allowed to develop. Depression in the mother is particularly disadvantageous at this time, when the basic task is to develop a strong attachment with the new baby. Severe depression removes mothers from their mothering functions, and consequently the amount of contact and the opportunity to build attachment are curtailed. Psychotherapeutic exploration during pregnancy of the above scenario can help prevent a severe depressive reaction.

Infants are also rendered vulnerable by the prepartum behavior of their mothers. Sleep disturbances, anxiety, depression, agitation, poor nutrition, intake of noxious substances, and general poor health of the woman, all interfere with optimal fetal development. Frequently, it is not only a lack of knowledge about birth and babies which heavily contributes to detrimental behaviors but psychodynamic factors. After appropriate psychotherapeutic intervention, it is often found that previously the client more or less knew what she "should" be doing, but had been unable to act accordingly.

For women with conflicts and/or problems, the opportunity to work such issues through in an appropriate manner is of enormous advantage. Socioeconomic debilities are also a risk factor, and breakdowns associated with pregnancy or childbirth have been found to be high for depressed and schizophrenic women (Stevens, 1971). Initial breakdowns during the first postpartum year have also been found to be extremely high (Wynne, 1984). Pregnancy is an excellent time for an intervention for the emotionally disturbed woman. She is more highly motivated, as well as more in need of emotional support, than she typically is. She is consequently more receptive to appropriate psychotherapeutic contacts.

PREGNANCY-ORIENTED PSYCHOTHERAPY

Interventions should start during pregnancy in order to deal with these emotionally difficult issues that otherwise may affect subsequent events (see Appendix D, "Guide to Treatment Planning"). Pregnancy-oriented psychotherapy also addresses: the excacerbation of psychopathology during the puerperium; the development by the woman of delusions involving the fetus; conflicts concerning the continuation of the pregnancy; fears concerning parturition; conflicts concerning the disposition of the baby; unrealistic expectations in relation to the baby; the intrapsychic meaning and psychotic distortions of being a mother; the exploration of the existence of a network of significant others (next of kin, family, friends, neighbors, and community agencies); and the development of a therapeutic alliance that will be in place in time for the presence of the infant.

When the therapist works with the mother to resolve conflicts to the extent possible, to prepare the mother for the reality of the advent of the infant, to prevent or diminish the psychopathological reaction to the pain of childbirth, these efforts act to diminish the unrealistic expectations the mother may have of herself, the infant, the father, and significant others. There is limited time in which to accomplish these specific therapeutic goals during pregnancy. It is therefore useful for the therapist to channel the therapy to specific foci which are important for the client. In actual practice, it is sometimes necessary to introduce topic areas, for example, in order to ensure that the individual deals with these prior to the birth of the baby.

To the extent to which significant conflicts are resolved and specific treatment goals are accomplished, the mother is protected from fear, anxiety, and depression. Also, the infant is protected from the mother's reactions to these forces and potential interferences with her ability to interact naturally and positively with the infant. The best interests of the child-to-be are therefore served significantly by the specific pregnancy-oriented therapy in a truly preventive manner.

SOME QUESTIONS AND ANSWERS

Why is pregnancy-oriented psychotherapy focused on issues of the infant-to-be?

In individual psychotherapy, generally there is no particular focus on specific issues. Rather, the issues that are taken up are what predominate in the psyche of the individual who is coming for help: those problems that are foremost, with a gradual working back to core issues, problems, and conflicts of that person. I consider pregnancy-oriented psychotherapy a quasi-crisis-oriented kind of intervention: no matter what the level of progress made in the psychotherapy, and the speed at which this is done, the baby will in fact be born within a certain period of time. It is a time-limited situation. Pregnancy-oriented psychotherapy, as such, comes to a halt with the birth of the baby. Therefore, the orientation and goals of pregnancy-oriented psychotherapy are not the restructuring of the personality of the pregnant woman in the therapy situation, unless this can be accomplished within the nine months or fewer available for the pregnancy-oriented psychotherapy. In many instances the psychotherapy does not start at the beginning of pregnancy but some time during the pregnancy period. At times, it may be quite late in the pregnancy. The time period available for the therapy varies but does not exceed nine months. In most instances it is not realistic to think of restructuring the personality during that period of time, or even to deal with the major issues pertinent to that individual's overall adjustment. Therefore, the approach is a focused one, specific to issues having to do with the state of pregnancy, the anticipation of the baby, and the birth process itself.

Why is it so important to have more optimal interaction between mother and baby from the earliest time possible?

There are fundamentally two reasons. First, the basic psychological structures, foundations, and reaction patterns are set into motion from the very beginning. The child has a great deal of flexibility in terms of how it will develop its psychological structures, functions, and behavior patterns. These become increasingly defined as the baby interacts with its world. Basically, it can be conceptualized as a kind of decision tree, in computer language, where one starts at one point and soon comes to rather specific decision points. Similarly, the structures of the baby are at first very general and become increasingly specific as it develops, depending upon what happens in the life of the child.

Second, the life-long pattern of interaction is set into motion from the earliest beginnings. Not only is the baby's internalized psychological structure (the *anlage*) set at the earliest times, but also the interaction pattern between mother and child. This pattern then influences the next steps of the manner of interaction between mother and child. For instance, an early positive interaction pattern will help the mother to expect positive actions and reactions from the baby and to take joy in this. The mother will then approach the baby with that anticipation and will tend to provide positive stimulation for the baby, such as nurturing, playfulness, emotional warmth, and so on. This in turn stimulates more positive actions and reactions on the part of the baby. In most cases the caretaker remains the same person, typically the mother. Therefore, the pattern set into motion from the very beginning continues to grow on itself throughout the developmental years of the child. That pattern has an opportunity to impact the child not only in the beginning but on a continuing basis.

How is it possible for a disturbed woman to tend to deny her pregnancy and remain apparently oblivious to it?

In relation to all pregnancies, as to all life situations, there is a degree of ambivalence present: there are at the same time positive and negative feelings about being pregnant. There is, by definition, the presence of two forces, or valences, in this ambivalence. The strength of the positive and negative valences will determine the person's reaction of ambivalence. In most cases, when a woman is pregnant, if it is a wanted pregnancy, she will have a predominantly positive valence, even though there may be some negative feelings about it. On the other hand, in most instances, when the pregnancy is not wanted, there would be a predominantly negative valence. The probability is that there would also be some positive feelings about being pregnant. When the valences are extremely disproportionate, decisions about the pregnancy will be more easily conceptualized by the woman. The closer the valences come to each other, in other words, the more closely balanced the positive and negative valences are, the greater the conflicts. For example, Mrs. X has wanted to have a baby for many years. She became pregnant at a time when conflicts arose due to other things in the marriage situation. She might have both strong positive and negative feelings at the same time about being pregnant and be strongly conflicted. That such feelings are on a conscious level does not lessen the conflict; however, it is possible to examine the situation rationally and come to a decision as to what to do about it. On the other hand, when there is a strong conflict that is not within the awareness of the individual, it is not possible to deal with the conflict by using problem-solving techniques. When the conflict is embedded in other psychological stresses or conflicts, it may not be at a conscious level. In that case, the paradigm is the typical one for psychotherapeutic intervention. Therapy is needed in order for the person to be able to deal with the unconscious material and to resolve the conflict.

If the conflict remains unresolved, it can express itself in a denial of the pregnancy. This is a very difficult feat to accomplish, especially as the pregnancy continues, followed by the birth of a child. An alternative scenario is that the woman represses her negative feelings about the pregnancy, and in effect convinces herself that she has no such feelings. With repression, the unconscious, negative feelings may express themselves in a rejecting, hostile attitude toward the baby.

Why might a more seriously disturbed person have irrational fears of harming her fetus?

The more seriously disturbed person's inner conflicts and turmoil reflect stronger conflicts and anxieties, and also trace back to earlier years in her own development. There will have been a greater and more long-standing opportunity for her to have repressed her feelings. These feelings would be less available to conscious inspection. One of the most disturbing undesirable emotions is anger. When there is a need for repression, it is typically because the feelings are so strong they are considered destructive of the individual. Consequently, a very disturbed person may have very strong repressed hostile impulses. When this person is a mother-to-be, those impulses may be present in relation to the fetus.

For example, Mrs. Y has a generalized anger toward men, which has developed over time. The father of the baby does not welcome the baby. The patient tends to experience this as a rejection of herself. Her reaction encounters the substrata of anger and hostility. A flood of hostile feelings may surface. The fetus may be seen as the cause of her experienced anger and therefore become its object. Since the patient's feelings are intense and unacceptable to herself, she will work to repress them. They may then surface as fears of harming her fetus.

If, on the other hand, the conflicts have not been resolved, and the decision is to give birth to the baby, there will be other consequences. Typically, negative feelings about having the baby will be present. These will impact on the interaction between mother and child. At the extreme, negative feelings may well have an effect on the decision as to who will be the child's caretaker. There will be an impact on the entire life of the child and of the mother. Negative remains of the unresolved conflicts during pregnancy will influence her decision as to whether she assumes the caretaking/mothering role for her baby, gives the baby up for adoption or foster care, or opts for extensive day care. It will influence how she specifically resolves the living situation and care of the baby.

Why is it important to deal psychotherapeutically with fears concerning parturition?

For one thing, fear and anxiety increase the difficulty of childbirth and increase the anxiety around having the baby. If the individual is an emotionally disturbed person, it can also have the effect of exacerbating the symptoms. The reason for this is that, typically, in childbirth there is intolerable pain, which is in turn interpreted by the woman according to her psychodynamics. A typical reaction is that this is interpreted as punishment. This interpretation of pain can be prevented by preventive psychotherapeutic intervention specifically dealing with this issue, prior to parturition.

Many first admissions of women to mental hospitals follow the birth of a child. For less disturbed women, the exacerbations of symptoms would be increased anxiety, depression, and so on. Consequently, at the very time when the emotional armamentarium of the woman is most needed by another individual, the baby, she is least accessible to the child. Therefore, dealing with concerns around parturition is of great importance in cases where there is a psychological disturbance in the woman, and specifically in cases where there are fears in relation to parturition.

What is the importance of dealing with any unrealistic expectations in relation to the baby during the pregnancy?

It is often the case that the emotionally deprived pregnant woman, either consciously or unconsciously, has expectations of the baby which are unrealistic. A common expectation is that the baby will provide love and nurturance to the mother, who has been deprived of this all her life. This is unrealistic on the part of the mother because the baby is not initially equipped to give but only to take. In fact, it needs to develop within itself and within the relationship before the mother can gain a sense of being able to receive from the baby. The mother who expects to receive love from the newborn baby is setting herself up for a tremendous disappointment. The baby, being a demanding bundle of needs, rapidly ushers in this disappointment. Because of her disappointment in the baby, the mother tends to react with anger, possibly with rejection of the baby.

What is the importance of exploring the intrapsychic meanings and possible distortions about being a mother, psychotherapeutically?

Generally, the state of being a mother has the meaning to the female that she is now a fully grown adult, a person who is responsible and respected. In most instances a new mother will, to a large extent, be right in assuming that she is now fully grown and has the regard of others as a full adult. However, the teenager may well have the same expectation, yet not be confirmed by others in this way. She will then be disappointed and hurt in still being treated as a teenager, without necessarily realizing that this was her expectation. If this is not clarified and integrated by the young mother, then there will be anger toward the child for having "fooled her," for having led her astray.

For the disturbed mother who may have distorted ideas about her power over the baby, and/or the child's power over her, the disappointment would be a detrimental and possibly destructive element in her interaction with the child. Her most probable reaction would be one of anger.

Why would an emotionally disturbed person tend to have alienated his/her family of origin over the years?

The emotionally disturbed individual has needs that have long been unmet, which the individual is constantly striving to meet. For instance, the need to feel accepted by others is basic. Often the core problem is that of not having been accepted by the most important people in one's life. Typically, the parents and others in the primary environment during the early developmental years carry great importance. Since this need has not been met, the person will either defend against awareness of having the need, because it is so hurtful, or he/she might act out. That is, the individual might commit acts that express his/her need for acceptance. Doing poorly in school, getting into fights, or directly disobeying parents are all ways of expressing anger and also of getting attention from parents. Acting out does accomplish getting their attention, but this attention is negative and makes the parents angry. If the child has utilized repression, these needs will tend to show themselves in symptom formation. For example, the child might develop phobic symptoms. Phobic symptoms have a secondary effect. They are not only extremely disturbing to the individual, but in addition they are often very disturbing to the people around him/her. These symptoms may interfere with the family's functioning. For instance, if the person is afraid of the dark he/she may never be willing to go into a dark space. Or suppose there is a fear of trains: these may be avoided, thereby keeping the family from taking trips on trains. Symptoms are usually annoying to others. The family is annoyed by the emotionally disturbed child. As the child grows up and is non-functional as an adult, he/she cannot earn money. Now the family will be additionally drained. They may have to support that family member and take care of his/her financial commitments, including treatment. Very frequently, the family that has been taking care of the emotionally disturbed person for many years is, at minimum, irritated, and maximally has severed the relationship.

Why is the family's alienation from the disturbed mother-to-be so devastating?

The pregnant woman is relatively debilitated. At the time of delivery she is incapacitated. The experience of the woman is one of being more vulnerable. Therefore it is natural to be, and to feel, more dependent during this time. This typically may go unnoticed when there are loving and caring people who surround the mother-to-be and whom she feels she can depend upon and feel comfortable with. She may not even be aware of her feelings of dependency. Similarly, an emotionally healthy person who is alone during the pregnancy period may also be able to supply enough comfort for herself and depend upon herself to, more or less, make up for the lack of other support people. This is actually a rare situation because an emotionally healthy person will probably not have alienated her family and friends. There will likely be some degree of relationship and emotional support available to her from others.

The emotionally disturbed mother, on the other hand, not only has chronically unmet emotional needs, but these are excacerbated by this time when dependency is highlighted. Consequently her need to have her needs met is greater. She will experience these lacks more keenly. If she is sufficiently repressed, these forces will remain under control. They will, however, tend to surface as symptoms. During pregnancy they will be expressed in relation to the baby-to-be.

How does severe depression tend to remove the mother from her mothering functions?

Depression, by definition, has the behavioral effect of reducing the activity and reactivity level. If the depressed person is a mother of a baby, then the activity and reactivity in relation to the baby would be diminished. That is, she will tend to have less interaction with the baby. She will be less animated and less playful in her interaction. She will have less joy in her interactions with the baby. In severe depression, she may just leave the baby in the crib. She may either go about her business, not paying attention to the baby, or she may be immobilized by her depression and do nothing. She may just sit, or may lie in bed, or sleep a great deal. In such states she may not react to the demands of her child. She is lacking sufficient energy and/or interest to take care of her child. This is particularly devastating in a one-parent household. If there are more people in the household, the lack of interaction with the mother could, at least in part, be compensated for by others. In fact, it has been typical in our society for others in the household to have taken care of the baby. There is, however, an increasing number of one-parent households. The number of mothers who put their children at risk due to their depression is increasing. The children thereby have a less than optimal start in terms of their own development. The children will tend to have limited feelings of relatedness to others, feel a lack of power, and have a poor sense of self. They feel that they lack the power to influence others to effect getting their needs met.

Why is the pregnancy period an excellent time for psychothera-peutic intervention for the emotionally disturbed woman?

The finding is that all women who are either expecting a child or have a baby want the best for their child. That is, all women have an intrinsic interest in seeing their child do well in life. For the woman who, in her own perception, has not done well in her own life, the anticipated birth of a new child is typically experienced as another opportunity for the mother to do well through the child. That is, since the child is experienced as an extended part of herself, the child's happiness and success in life is seen, in a way, as her own happiness and accomplishment. There is an anticipa-tion of a new lease on life for the pregnant woman, especially for the woman who does not feel she has fulfilled her needs or ambitions. She is more highly motivated and open to psychotherapeutic intervention during this period of pregnancy because she sees this as a new beginning. With therapy, she learns to recognize that this beginning can be different and can be an improvement over her own life.

Another reason for being more amenable to psychotherapeutic interven-tion during the period of pregnancy is because of the woman's need for emotional support and increased dependency that is heightened during pregnancy. The person with the greatest dependency needs is frequently well defended in relation to them. That is, she may not be aware of them and so not express them directly. This is because these needs have not been met, and the person has developed the expectation that they will not be met. Allowing herself to experience these dependency needs is a painful experience, with the expectation of their not being met. However, in the pregnancy, there is a natural increase in dependency needs and needs for emotional support. If this support is offered, as it is in pregnancy-oriented psychotherapy, and dependency needs are allowed to be experienced and expressed without punishment and with resultant nurturant reactions on the part of the therapist, the individual becomes more available to thera-peutic intervention. This is a prime time, and a very appropriate time, for psychotherapeutic interventions for the disturbed mother-to-be.

Why is it so important to deal psychotherapeutically with the development of delusions involving the fetus during pregnancy?

It is best always to deal with delusions before they become crystallized. Delusions are symptoms that form when the anxiety level gets too high in the individual to be tolerable. If, during the period of the development of the delusions, the anxiety level can be diminished through psychotherapeutic means, the formation of delusions can be modified. In the case of the pregnant woman, a delusion in relation to the fetus can actually be caught in the process of development. Since this is a new happening in the life of the person, there is first of all the possibility of preventing the formation of the delusion. Second, it is extremely important to do so. Once a delusion in relation to the fetus is set, it will probably tend to remain, even after the baby's birth. This can lead to a situation that can put the baby at risk. For instance, suppose the mother's delusion is that the baby is evil. The reaction by the mother could either be to be afraid of, or to be aggressive toward, the baby, or both.

What is the importance of dealing psychotherapeutically with conflicts concerning the continuation of the pregnancy?

Conflict concerning continuation of the pregnancy produces a good deal of pressure on a pregnant woman. She knows that she has a limited time during which any resolution of that conflict can be made. After a certain time, the options are essentially gone. Not having the opportunity to work through this conflict is always detrimental. If the woman decides to terminate the pregnancy without the utilization of pregnancy-oriented psychotherapy, there are typically regrets. There will also be a need to replace that pregnancy with another one. This is most frequently at an unconscious level. If conflicts have not been resolved, or needs have not been met, or situations have not been changed by the time of the next pregnancy, then the same dilemma has a tendency to be repeated.

3

The Necessary Structures, Foundations, and Conceptual Framework for Focused and Effective Preventive Psychotherapy: Four Types of Severely Emotionally Disturbed Mothers and Their Mothering

To be effective and successful in both treatment and prevention requires a clear and basic framework of theory and concept. Without this framework, effective results cannot be achieved efficiently and the interventions cannot be as effectively taught.

This chapter describes how positive outcomes have been achieved following a clear theoretical framework. It provides the therapist a preface to a focused conceptual foundation and structure upon which to begin to plan and build effective prenatal and postnatal treatment and positive outcomes.

This chapter sets forth the conceptual framework for dyadic psychotherapy. Based upon the author's findings and observation, four types of the most severely disturbed and psychotic mothers are operationally defined. This chapter describes resultant types of mothering that are found. The significance, characteristics, impact, the meaning of fear, anxiety, depression, and defenses are noted in terms of: Type 1, Schizophrenic mothers; Type 2, Paranoid Schizophrenic mothers; Type 3, Bipolar mothers; and Type 4, mothers with Major Depression. This chapter begins to lay out a foundation and the structure of theory for specific, appropriate, and differential interventions which will be discussed fully in later chapters.

By starting with the most extreme end of the spectrum of psychopathology, one acquires some basic observations and findings that will apply, in various degrees, to the less disturbed and to the "normal" end of the scale.

The postpartum period is a prime time for psychotherapeutic intervention for parent and infant. Contact and relationship between baby and parent become the most important element in both worlds. The opportunity to form a therapeutic alliance is particularly strong and ensuing psychotherapy remarkably effective.

Once the baby arrives, child rearing harbors problems for all parents. For the normal mother, however, the task is predominantly rewarding. There is a great deal of satisfaction in watching and helping an infant grow and develop. The mother typically experiences intense joy in her closeness to and her love for the infant. A deeply satisfying interplay develops between mother and infant, typified by a good deal of contingent interaction in which the mother reacts to the baby and the baby reacts to the mother. In the emotionally disturbed parent, to the extent that these normal processes are interfered with, there is trouble in the nursery. The deeply satisfying nature of the interaction tends to ensure its occurrence in most cases. However, when the mother is very deeply disturbed, there tends to be a very profound interference.

It is clear that Mary, described in the first chapter, has had a dysfunctional family background. Presently she also has a non-nurturing family and a difficult living situation. It is not a surprise, therefore, that the manner in which she handles her baby might not be optimal. In dealing with her clinically, it would be tremendously advantageous to have an understanding of the basic internal forces that help to determine her behaviors, how these are expressed in mothering behaviors, and how these affect the emotional development of the infant. This understanding would allow the therapist to have a theoretical framework to help target psychotherapeutic interventions. Targeted interventions help to attain efficiency in the therapeutic process. This is particularly important in work with infants because of their own rapid development and because of the development of interactional styles between mother and infant.

In general, people are able to interact, work, and play in a natural, spontaneous manner, at the same time taking into account the many opportunities and limitations the realities of their lives place upon them.

There are *states* and *traits* that create problems in living. A *state* may be defined as a condition that exists at this time and impacts on the individual's functioning. A *trait* may be defined as a condition that is an enduring aspect of the personality. Three basic *states* that interfere with the ability to function well are fear, anxiety, and depression. When these *states* persist, they tend to become *traits*, and defenses are gradually organized by the individual to deal with them. These become negative factors influencing behavior.

THE DIFFERENCE BETWEEN FEAR AND ANXIETY

A person faced with a ferocious dog running toward him/her will experience fear. Anxiety, on the other hand, is typically associated with negative emotions or frustrations. For instance, the inability to solve a problem or deal with a situation generates anxiety. A loss, for example, the loss of a loved one, also tends to generate anxiety. Concomitant happenings may also kindle anxiety by associations, so that a song heard at the same time a trauma was experienced will tend to trigger anxiety when heard again later on. For example, if fear was engendered by a ferocious dog and at the same time a particular song was playing, there would be fear of the dog but anxiety in relation to the song.

Typically, fear has a specific object that one is consciously afraid of, whereas anxiety may occur without an awareness of its source.

Depression is a state that occurs when the individual feels helpless, that one has no impact on others, on situations, or on having one's needs met.

These three states create typical general reactions.

THREE BASIC STATES

1. *Fear.* The natural reaction to fear is flight. When physical flight is not possible, it may be expressed in other avoidant behavior (such as avoidance of eye contact). When fear becomes intense, panic sets in, which can result in freezing behavior (e.g., standing or sitting very still).
2. *Anxiety.* Anxiety basically functions to distort one's reactions. It is disorganizing (Grubler, 1957).
3. *Depression.* Depression's basic effect is to inhibit one's behavior. It slows or eliminates the individual's reactions.

When fear, anxiety, and/or depression are severe and endure, they tend to become traits. Their painful nature stimulates the individual to develop coping techniques. These serve the purpose of diminishing the pain. These do allow the individual some control and therefore ability to function. When these coping mechanisms are inflexible and not under conscious control, they are called defenses.

Defenses

Defenses are an effort to control the states of fear, anxiety, and depression; to cope, to adjust behavior, and thereby to approach the normal or

Table 3.1
Negative Factors and Their Direct Effects on Behavior

Negative Factors	*Direct Effects on Behavior*
Fear	Avoidance
	Flight
	Freezing
Anxiety	Distortion
	Disorganization
Depression	Inhibition of behavior (slowing or elimination of reactions)
Defenses	Attempts to cope and to approach normal reactions may evolve into the form of symptoms of psychopathology.

natural (Grubler, 1957). When the states are severe and enduring, symptoms of psychopathology evolve from the defenses.

Defenses, once developed, tend to take on a functional autonomy and to become part of the typical functioning of the person. Because of the negative quality of these states and traits (Beck, 1967; Spielberger, 1972) and of the defenses, they will hereafter be referred to as negative factors that influence behavior. The influences of these negative factors are listed below and are summarized in Table 3.1.

Emotionally disturbed individuals have various mixes of these negative factors that influence behavior. The specific mix is typical per diagnosis.

TYPE 1: THE SCHIZOPHRENIC MOTHER, PREDOMINANTLY NON-PARANOID TYPE

Schizophrenics are highly fearful, are also anxious, and have developed a variety of symptoms. For example, they may have hallucinations and delusions. However, if they are essentially non-paranoid (Garmezy and Phipps-Yonas, 1984), they have not developed the tightest of defenses. They will probably also show depression to some extent. The degree of depression can vary greatly.

Consequently we find that the mother who falls into the Type 1 category will be typified by the following behavioral reactions: avoidance of contact with other people (fear); distortions, bizarre behaviors (anxiety); some tendency to inhibit reactions (depression); and possibly a range of other behavioral symptoms such as obsessive-compulsive symptoms, phobias, hallucinations, and delusions (see Table 4.1).

Fears

As a reaction to her fears, the Type 1 schizophrenic mother will tend to avoid close contact in relation to her infant. This avoidance will be exhibited in many significant ways such as: holding the child as little as possible; a lack of molding of mother and infant when she holds the baby; facing the baby away from her; holding the baby stiffly; and putting the baby across her lap while she is sitting, giving the impression of an object rather than a baby (the "log effect"). Avoidance of close contact will also be exhibited by: gaze avoidance (the mother will not look in the baby's eyes); a lack of auditory stimulation (the mother will tend not to talk to her baby, nor sing or make other sounds such as baby talk); a lack of vestibular stimulation (the mother will tend not to move the baby such as in rocking, cradling, or other gentle holding movements which would stimulate the vestibular, inner ear, mechanism).

Anxiety

As a reaction to her anxiety, the Type 1 schizophrenic mother will have distorted behaviors in relating to her infant. She will tend to have unrealistic perceptions and expectations of the baby. The specifics will vary by individual. She may, for instance, expect the infant to be much more mature and therefore be able to feed itself; and/or know the mother's needs and satisfy them, and so on. The inability of the infant to fulfill these expectations may engender anger and/or depression, which in turn could result in physical abuse or neglect, or lesser variations thereof.

Depression

As a result of her depression, the Type 1 mother, in relation to her infant, will tend to interact less with her baby, be unresponsive to the child's needs, and have less enthusiasm and interest in the child.

Defenses

The results of other symptoms of the Type 1 mother on behavior toward her baby will vary according to the specific symptoms she has evolved. For instance, obsessive-compulsive symptoms may express themselves in tightly controlling the intake of food by the infant, which may result in deficiency or overfeeding; or, for example, phobias that may result in severe overprotectiveness of the baby, perhaps resulting in dressing the baby in vastly too many layers of clothing. If there are sexual disturbances, these may show themselves in sexually abusive behavior. If substance abuse is involved, neglect of the infant may result.

TYPE 2: THE PARANOID SCHIZOPHRENIC MOTHER

The paranoid schizophrenic individual has basically the same core structure as the non-paranoid. This type of mother, however, has developed a tight defensive system of paranoid ideation. She has been able to project fears, bad impulses, and anxieties-distortions onto others. To the extent to which she is successful in the projection, she is free of fears and anxieties. Since the levels of fear and anxiety are high, it requires a tight system for this control. As a result, the paranoid schizophrenic individual may often be more functional than the non-paranoid person. She also tends to suffer less from depression. The predominant symptom here is the paranoid ideation.

In relation to her baby, the Type 2 paranoid schizophrenic mother will display less avoidant behavior. In fact, if the paranoid system is working well, she will approach the norm in interacting with her baby, and even perhaps surpass the norm, producing overstimulation (see Table 4.2). Consequently the Type 2 paranoid-schizophrenic mother will be typified by the following behaviors.

Fears

In the Type 2 paranoid schizophrenic mother, fear will tend to be handled dynamically through denial. She may therefore tend not to display avoidant behavior. In fact, the paranoid schizophrenic mother is typified by the opposite. There is intrusive behavior. She does not avoid the infant, but rather intrudes herself onto the infant. Nevertheless, underneath her paranoid defenses, the fear remains. Consequently, her contact with her infant will fail to be on target. She may hold the baby, but will hold it uncomfortably, perhaps too much. She will look at the baby and make eye contact, but this may be at times very intense, and at other times be avoidant, or her behavior may have other irregularities. She may talk too much, or too intrusively to the baby, or she may talk to the baby in an unmodulated voice. Her rocking, holding, cradling, carrying, and other movements of her baby may be unrelenting, intensive, erratic, forceful, or show other unpleasant characteristics. There can be interferences with this behavior. For example, the effects of the use of psychotropic medication acts as a tranquilizer, and serves to reduce the general energy level and tendency to action by the mother. This might lessen the above behaviors. Or she may be inadequately defended, and consequently display avoidant behavior.

Depression

The Type 2 mother may be concomitantly depressed and therefore display a diminished activity level with lower consequent levels of the above behaviors. The "log effect" (baby across the lap, immobile) may therefore be a result, though it is not otherwise typical of the Type 2 mother.

Anxiety

The Type 2 paranoid schizophrenic mother may be well enough defended from her anxiety to have little generalized distortions in her behavior in relation to her infant. She may be able to interact with the baby in an apparently normal manner. She may study what is expected of an infant and try to apply this knowledge to mothering. However, the interactions will be rigid and will tend to be stereotyped. A lack of flexibility will show itself in the rigidity of timing, manner, and emotions related to mother-baby interactions. Consequently, the mother will be overcontrolling of the infant. She may seem to be overprotective and possessive. She may feel that she does not want others near her baby and will tend to keep the child apart from others.

Defenses

Since the predominant defense is paranoid ideation, the behavior resulting from this defense depends upon the content of the ideation. If the paranoid system of the mother does not involve the baby, the resultant behaviors may not significantly impinge upon the baby, or may do so only indirectly. If, however, the paranoid ideation involves the baby, there are direct results. That is, if her voices tell the mother to treat the baby in a certain way, or to harm it, or to neglect it, she will be driven to do so. The intensity of the thought will determine whether or not the mother acts upon it. For example, in the case of a mother whose voices told her to go to the zoo and feed her baby to the lions, she took her infant to the zoo, but fortunately did not follow through in attempting to feed her infant to the lions.

The typical behavior of the Type 2 paranoid schizophrenic is intrusive overstimulation, overprotectiveness, and overpossessiveness. If the mother's delusions involve the child, there are dangers that the mother could be abusive or neglectful.

TYPE 3: THE BIPOLAR MOTHER

The bipolar Type 3 mother is devastatingly depressed. This is her predominant symptom. If she is unipolar, her state will vary between severe depression and a more even state. If she is bipolar, she will vary between extremely severe depression and degrees of mania. The basic dynamic is a sense of worthlessness (Gochman, 1985) developed in early childhood, which is based in a sense of helplessness (Seligman, 1975), hopelessness, and depression. The sense of helplessness tends to result in despairing of the attempt to take the initiative in one's own life. The desperate hope is that someone else will meet one's needs. There is therefore a profound continuing sense of dependency on others. With this profound dependency need comes anger at feeling so deeply dependent and at the object of this dependency. The person is consequently hopeless of ever feeling adequate. As Gochman (1985) has indicated, the feeling of being unable to exert an effect upon others, to have no impact on one's parent or caretaker to have needs met, inevitably raises the question in the individual's mind as to what is the reason for this. The readily available answer for attribution is that one must be worthless. This attribution of worthlessness, once developed, becomes highly intransigent to change, and remains relatively impervious to new experience.

The effort of the Type 3 bipolar patient is to gain some small sense of self-worth. The patient is therefore continually trying to prove herself, and is preoccupied with making an impression on others in order to do so. The effort cannot succeed, however, because no success can really be accepted by the person as evidence of self-worth to counter the basic sense of worthlessness. Instead, successes are rationalized. For instance, getting good grades "is only because I'm smart"; being a good dancer "is only because I had lessons." No indication of success functions to satisfy the need to feel worthwhile. Typically the Type 3 bipolar depressed are not inordinately fearful or anxious. The direct effect of this type of depression on behavior is to inhibit it, to diminish reactions. The direct effect of hypomania on behavior is disinhibition, to amplify and accelerate reactions and behavior. The activity level of the Type 3 psychotically depressed mother, at any given time, depends upon the present state of her depression or mania. This varies across time. Consequently, the behavior of a given individual will appear very different at different times. The one constant across time is the continuous significant effect of the sense of worthlessness. It results in a preoccupation with self-enhancement and consequent lack of intrinsic interest in others.

The effect of Type 3 bipolar depression on the mother's interaction with her infant varies with the state of the mother, but also maintains a consistency. As the mother varies as to her activity level, her behavior with the infant will vary accordingly. During a hypomanic phase she may not have the patience to care for her child and may try to have someone else care for it, or may abandon it, or may put the child in danger because of her high level of activity. For instance, she may ask a stranger to watch her children and then disappear for hours or days. During severe depression the Type 3 mother may neglect the infant because of depressed interest and/or energy in relation to the baby.

When these states are less pronounced, the effect of the Type 3 mother's sense of worthlessness will tend to be clearer. Since she is seeking some sense of worth, she will try to enhance herself in an effort to accomplish this. For instance, if she has the idea of being a "good mother," she will try to play that role. However, since her interest is not so much focused on the infant's well-being, but rather on her self-enhancement, she will tend to do "mothering" when it meets her needs rather than the infant's needs. She will be particularly concerned when another person, whose opinion is important to the mother, is present. The effort is to have that person see her as a "good mother." The interaction with her baby will therefore be non-contingent (Ferster & Skinner, 1957), that is, non-contingent on the momentary needs and demands of the infant (see Table 4.3).

TYPE 4: THE MOTHER WITH MAJOR DEPRESSION

The Type 4 mother with major depression appears and is extremely depressed. She takes little pleasure nor has interest in herself or in what is happening around her. She may have preoccupations with death and/or suicide. She is not able to function in her daily life, to care for herself adequately, or to care for her family.

The basic dynamics of the Type 4 mother are severe guilt feelings and a sense of "helplessness" (Seligman, 1975). It is not the basic helplessness of the bipolar, who has incorporated the experience of being unable to produce an effect upon others in his/her demands to have his/her needs met. Rather, persons with major depression feel that they do not deserve to have their needs met because of their guilt. They have an unrealistic sense of having the power to have detrimental effects upon others. The helplessness is consequently, in a sense, self-imposed (psychodynamically). They are not allowed to help themselves because they are guilty of terrible impulses.

In the Type 4 mother, the causes of problems are attributed to herself, with a concomitant well-ingrained sense of being unable to do anything to alleviate the problems. Problems are seen as insurmountable. Support people are subjectively depended upon to deal with problems. This is the case even when she is the one who in reality is the functioning partner, for example, the main breadwinner of the family. There may be resultant resentment and anger, with consequent increased guilt feelings. The loss of such a support person by the Type 4 mother is therefore experienced as a loss of the ability to cope, being helpless, and is being the guilty party in having caused the loss. If the loss is due to the death of the support person, this tends to be experienced as overwhelming (guilt and helplessness), and decompensation may result.

The effect on the Type 4 mother's interaction with her infant is to diminish them. She will tend to sit passively, quietly watching her child. The mother will tend to avoid physical contact with her child, generally displaying a tentativeness. It is as though she makes an effort to avoid doing anything that might alienate the child from her. The mother tends to use what energies she can garner to pay attention to her child (rather than to other adults who are present, as in the bipolar mother). She hopes that the child will not reject her (see Table 4.4).

SOME QUESTIONS AND ANSWERS

Why are targeted interventions important in dyadic psychotherapy for mother and infant?

Dyadic psychotherapy for mother and infant is also a quasi-crisis-oriented intervention, as is pregnancy-oriented psychotherapy. Here there is also a time element involved. The interactions of mother and child need to be age-appropriate. Dyadic psychotherapeutic intervention cannot run on its own timetable, but rather on that of the baby's developmental stages. The psychotherapeutic interventions must be appropriate to the level at which the baby's development is at the present time, as well to the next anticipated developmental phases. The psychotherapy needs to be targeted to relate to the developmental phases of the infant.

If anxiety is a natural reaction to frustrating situations, why is it problematic?

Let us say that someone is in a learning situation and fails to learn effectively. This frustration engenders anxiety. The anxiety will, under ordinary circumstances, be at a tolerable level to the person. Usually the person can utilize this anxiety as a kind of energy to propel him/her to try harder in the learning process. However, let us say there is a premium on learning this task, and there is enormous pressure to learn. The anxiety level may then be excessive. Consequently, it is the degree of anxiety which will determine its effect. At lower levels it is a help to learning, while at high levels it is a detriment. At any given time, there is typically some degree of anxiety in all of us, because we are frustrated in little ways as we go through our day. In a child who is inundated in frustration, not being able to cope with the home situation, there will be a buildup of anxiety. When this anxiety becomes overwhelming, it tends to interfere with the functioning of that individual, so that perception, cognitive functions, learning, and body movement, and so on will be affected. These changes will impact his/her interactions with the people he/she comes in contact with. Mental functions will be affected, such as the ability to concentrate and to perform in the conceptual realm.

In addition to fear having a specific object, what are some of the other characteristics of fear?

Fear is experienced on a conscious level. That is, the person knows what the object of the fear is, for example, a person, an animal, a situation. There is an awareness in relation to fear.

Another characteristic of fear is that there is a response to it. In other words, the person has specific responses to fears. The reaction is basically either fight or flight. In its simplest format, whether to fight or run away is determined by the person's perception of his or her ability to fight the object of the fear, that is, who is stronger. If the person sees him/herself as stronger, he/she will fight; if the person sees him/herself as weaker, he/she will fly. This is the natural reaction to fear. It is also the rational reaction to fear, and serves to protect one's own integrity. The characteristics of fear are that it has a specific object on a conscious level and there are behavioral reactions to it.

What are some of the characteristics of anxiety?

Anxiety does not have an object. There is not a particular person, animal, or situation that generates the anxiety in the individual, but rather the frustration is generated in dealing with these or in meeting one's own

needs. This may occur in conflict situations where two opposite behavioral reactions are stimulated which are incompatible, and where
there is no solution that the individual can fathom. The frustration in this
will create anxiety. Another characteristic of anxiety is that it is not
within the realm of awareness. Anxiety is generated as a reaction to the
frustration. The person experiences the anxiety only secondarily, after
the anxiety has been generated. The person is not necessarily aware of
the connection between the anxiety and its cause, the frustration. A
characteristic of anxiety is that since the connection to its source is not
within awareness, there is typically no ready behavioral reaction to it.
This creates confusion and additional anxiety, so that it tends to feed
upon itself.

What are some of the characteristics of depression?

Basically, it is the author's theoretical construct that depression results
from a sense of powerlessness to have one's needs met. One such type of
situation is when there is a loss of a person or object which is important
to the individual, for instance, as in the death of a loved one. The person's
experience is that he/she is powerless to bring the loved one back into
his/her life and therefore powerless to meet his/her emotional needs in that
relationship.

What are some of the coping mechanisms that are under conscious control?

The coping mechanisms under conscious control are those that most
people use in their everyday life: the rational process of analyzing a
situation and looking at all the factors involved, the goals and objectives
involved, making a decision as to how best to handle the situation, giving
weight and priority to factors that play a part in the situation, and thereby
coming to a decision, or perhaps a series of decisions, as to what to do.
If part of the problem involves a lack of skills or knowledge, the decision
may also involve a decision to learn certain things. Learning is a coping
mechanism. Ways of interacting with people are mechanisms that we use
all the time. That is, positive ways of interacting, ways of avoiding
disturbing the other person, and thereby getting the best results for
oneself, are coping devices that we have learned and that we use on a
conscious level. Characteristically, coping mechanisms, which are conscious, are flexible. Since we look at the situation consciously, we
maintain an openness to what might work best or what is most appropriate. Therefore, there is flexibility in the choice of behavioral
reactions to the situation.

What are some of the defenses that are used to protect against anxiety?

Repression, for instance, is a major defense mechanism which in effect serves to keep excessively painful thoughts, memories, or feelings out of consciousness. Denial is closely akin to it. This defense functions to deny, and thereby remove from awareness, that this problem area, emotion, or affective state is present. When a feeling, emotion, thought, or tendency to act is completely unacceptable to the person, defensive projection is sometimes used. The person feels that someone else has the feeling which really emanates from him/herself. In that way the person feels that the people around them are noxious rather than he/she. These are some of the examples.

How does avoidance work in dealing with fear?

Avoidance of the feared object can very well function protectively for the individual. For instance, if there is a fear of a particular dog, then staying away from that dog is an effective way of coping with that fear. However, when the fear becomes generalized, let us say to all animals, then the defense would have difficulty in functioning well because that would mean that all animals would need to be avoided in order to deal with the fear. This would tend to circumscribe the life of the individual. If the object of the fear is, for example, mathematics, and the defense is avoidance, then this could pose a particular problem for children. It would keep the child from exposure to mathematics, keeping the child from learning it, and thereby keep the child from overcoming the reason for its fear. The same would be true in interpersonal relations. The problem with avoidance is that it serves to remove the person from the feared object and thereby keep the person from possibly finding a way of overcoming the fear.

How does freezing function as a defense against fear?

It is observed in some animals that they will freeze when they are threatened by a larger animal. For instance, it can be noted in frogs and reptiles; when they feel there is danger, they will hold completely still for long periods of time. It functions as a defense for them in reducing their visibility because of the lack of movement. In the person who freezes in reaction to fear, this is perhaps a carryover from lower phylogenetic levels. In situations of aggression, such as war, keeping completely still does function as a defense. However, the psychological defense of freezing is not on a conscious level, but is a complete incapacitation of the person. It is probable that the basic mechanisms are the same, however. The results are typically not desirable. For instance, stage fright is to the detriment of the actor. Freezing in "test anxiety" is to the detriment of the student.

How is it that there is distortion and disorganization as a result of anxiety?

With very high levels of anxiety most people have experienced themselves as "unable to think." The anxiety is experienced as disorganizing. This is true in learning experiments as well, where high anxiety reduces learning ability. The distortion due to high levels of anxiety is also noted in studies of size perception (e.g., Grubler, 1957). Perception and the cognitive processes do not function in a regular way under the extraordinary conditions of high anxiety.

Why are defenses brought into play?

They are brought into play to deal with the states of fear, anxiety, and depression. When these states are at a high level, any one of them, or a combination of them, are experienced as intolerable by the individual, and consequently the intensity needs to be lessened. Defenses serve that purpose. This enables the individual to continue to function, even though perhaps it is at a different level, which is a compromised level.

Are schizophrenics highly fearful?

Schizophrenics are typified by excessively high levels of fear. They have not developed adequate levels of feelings of security during their developmental years to allow them to develop a self-concept with adequately firm boundaries to establish themselves as individuals separate and apart from others. It is my belief that throughout their development they are distracted by the fear they experience, interfering with the development of an adequate self-concept. They are fearful for the very integrity of their existence.

Are schizophrenics highly anxious?

It is the author's belief that there are two basic reasons why schizophrenics are highly anxious. In their interactions with their caretakers, from the earliest times of their development, their emotional needs have not been met adequately enough to satisfy them, thereby leaving them in a state of frustration. Second, because of their high levels of fear, they have not been able to function adequately enough so as to have their emotional needs met, again resulting in high levels of frustration. In consequence there is a great deal of anxiety present which tends to be continuously amplified due to frustrations in their lives. This high level of frustration, and consequent anxiety, has the effect of creating distortions in their perceptions and in their thinking process. Because of its high level, anxiety is extremely disruptive to the schizophrenic, which then creates further anxiety and other problems in symptom formation. Hallucinations are frequent symptoms of choice for the schizophrenic. These symptoms utilize the anxiety and make it possible for the person to regain some degree of equilibrium, though at a different level of adjustment, that is, an unrealistic one.

Why does the Type 1 schizophrenic mother avoid contact with other people?

The Type 1 schizophrenic person has learned through experience to be afraid of other people in early developmental years. He/she will generalize this fear to people in general, and will as a consequence tend to keep at a distance from other people. The Type 1 schizophrenic has not been able to develop adequate defenses to enable him/her to seek contact with others.

What are some types of perceptual distortions or bizarre behaviors in the Type 1 schizophrenic?

These distortions and behaviors may take many forms. For instance, the professional passing by the patient has been taken for her mother and been addressed in that way. Or the patient walks very carefully, keeping a distance from others. Another patient, in reading the newspaper, reads only peripheral items such as page numbers. Another patient may sit very still for long periods of time, just staring straight ahead. These are just some specific examples. Distortions and bizarre behaviors can take almost any form.

What are some of the symptoms of Type 1 schizophrenic reaction?

The symptoms may include delusions and hallucinations. However, they may also include an array of other symptoms. Obsessive-compulsive symptoms may be present, usually at the extreme, such as turning the water fountain on three times prior to taking a drink from it, gathering fuzzballs and little bits of string and keeping them in a safe place. Such symptoms may also include phobias, which are unrealistic fears, so that the patient may be on the lookout in order to avoid the object of the phobia. The symptoms may be fairly loose or be systematized. They may also include the typical symptoms of the subcategories of schizophrenia. Extreme symptoms are rarely seen today because of the use of psychotropic medications, which have the effect of tending to lessen the expression of these symptoms.

What does it mean that the Type 2 paranoid schizophrenic individual may often be more functional than the non-paranoid Type 1 person?

If the anxiety and fear of the individual are sufficiently controlled by the tight paranoid symptoms, the individual will be able to act in many ways as most other people do. They may be able to carry on a conversation, perform given tasks, be well groomed, and generally project an appearance that belies their severe psychopathological state. With a tightly systematized paranoid schizophrenic, sometimes only when the specific delusion is touched upon is there a realization of the severity of the psychopathology.

In relation to the Type 3 bipolar, how is the person's sense of helplessness developed?

According to the writer, the sense of helplessness is developed through non-contingent interactions. For instance, the baby is hungry and cries, the mother does not provide food at that time. Letting the mother know of the hunger does not lead to meeting those needs. The baby thereby learns that it cannot effect having its needs met. Later, when language emerges, the child speaks to the mother and the mother doesn't respond, or makes some unrelated comment. Another example: the toddler falls, hurting him/herself and comes to the mother; the mother pays no attention or makes an irrelevant comment, not meeting the emotional needs of the child to be soothed at that time. This same mother may, when she needs physical contact, take the child and cuddle it with "love." If the child is not receptive at that moment, it may struggle to loosen itself to get away from the mother. The mother will tend not to pay attention to this because she is busy trying to meet her own needs. Non-contingent interactions engender a sense of helplessness.

How is it that the child tends to attribute the reason for the sense of helplessness to him/herself?

At the time that the child develops language abilities, another phenomenon will happen. The thinking process/conceptual development is also taking place at this time. Once the child starts to conceptualize, he/she also starts to ask the question "why?" This question is typically posed by children in relation to many things. The child will also question the reason for being made to feel helpless. "Why does mommy not respond to my crying?" The inevitable answer to this question, in the child who has developed a sense of helplessess, is that "it must be because I, myself, am no good." Restated: "I cannot get mommy to listen to me, so I must be worthless," or "I am worthless and so mommy doesn't listen to me." Once the self-attribution of worthlessness is well cemented into the personality, it is not amenable to change.

Why is an individual's self-attribution of worthlessness not amenable to change?

The author posits that persons who suffer from a bipolar disorder have made a basic assumption about themselves. That basic assumption is the self-attribution of worthlessness. That is, their basic belief about themselves is that they are worthless. All other aspects of their self-concept have this as their base. Since it is a basic assumption, it is not amenable to logic; a basic assumption cannot be changed by logic. The person will feel that any positive attributes or achievements do not negate his/her basic assumption of worthlessness, but rather that these positives exist despite the fact that he/she is worthless.

Why does the Type 3 psychotically depressed mother vary across time in her state of depression and mania?

The answer to this is not clear, however the author feels that, in the extreme, the sense of worthlessness is intolerable, as is the extreme of severe depression. There is an internal struggle to overcome the sense of worthlessness and to be energized in so doing. The person will try to attain the feeling of in fact being worthwhile. In the attempt to convince oneself, he/she will try to convince others, hoping to receive the reflection of his/her conviction. Mania has grandiose elements. The person will dress and/or act in a grandiose fashion. They may, in the extreme, feel that they are better than everyone. The author feels that the Type 3 bipolar is in the throes of such an intense struggle that he/she cannot modulate this counterreaction to the feeling of worthlessness. They overshoot the mark of a normal mood state. They will then go into the manic phase. This is typified by the kind of behavior that is understood to be in the service of proving themselves worthwhile or important.

Can the Type 3 bipolar mother ever care for her little child?

In fact, many do. That is, when the mother is in a less extreme state of depression or mania, when she approaches the average or norm in activity level, she will be able to take care of her child. Most frequently such a person is called upon to do so, and is the caretaker. The emotional impact of the non-contingent type of interaction will be felt by the baby in its emotional development. There are possible counteractions to the development of the feeling of worthlessness in the baby due to the non-contingent interactions with the mother. It requires the presence of another person who is important to the child, is loving, and does interact contingently. If simultaneous with the non-contingent interaction with the mother, the baby/young child experiences a consistent caretaker who loves the child and interacts with him/her in a way that helps the child to feel that he/she can have an impact on having his/her needs met by someone, though this may not be the mother, it will tend to negate the development of an assumption by the child that it is indeed worthless. The child needs to have sufficient amount of contact with the contingently interacting caretaker; he/she needs to be able to separate conceptually the non-contingent interactions with the mother from the contingent interactions with other people. That is, the child needs to feel that the problem is with the mother and not with him/herself. In that way the child can avoid developing the devastating life-long basic assumption about him/herself: the self-attribution of worthlessness.

How long does a major depressive episode last?

Usually a major depressive episode lasts no longer than about six months. There may be a repetition of such an episode, and it may last considerably longer. The timing of the birth of the baby and the age of the baby when this episode is present is critical to developmental issues for the baby. Typically, as the depression subsides, the mother returns to her previous level of functioning. The worst effects on the baby occur during the episode. If the episode(s) occur during the child's formative months and years, the effect upon the child can be profound (depending upon what countermeasures are taken to protect the child from these effects).

Why does the Type 4 mother with major depression tend to interact with her child by sitting quietly, avoiding physical contact with her child?

The mother with major depression feels that the child will reject her. This is the fear that lingers and permeates any potential interactions with her child. She avoids physical contact with her child because she is afraid that this will not be welcomed. She feels guilty about her impulses which generally have hostile-aggressive content. She is afraid that the child will not react positively to her. The possible rejection is also scary in that it will tend to create further depression in the mother. Frequently the mother does not have the courage to make an advance toward the child and so will sit passively and hope that the child will come to her and will display acceptance and love of her, being herself unable to begin this process. During the worst parts of the depressive episode, the mother may not be able to garner enough energy even to sit passively and watch the child. She may be too preoccupied with her thoughts, guilt feelings, and possibly obsessions, as well as fears about the terrible things that might happen to her.

4

A Conceptual Framework, Continued
Four Types of Infants: Their Behavior
as Effects of Four Types of Severely
Emotionally Disturbed Mothering

This chapter discusses specific parent impact upon the infant. It further outlines my fundamental findings and theoretical notions which lay the structure and foundation for successful therapeutic intervention. There are remarkable relationships found between disturbed mothers' very specific mothering behaviors and their impacts upon the infants' behavior and interactions.

Infants of the four types of severely emotionally disturbed mothers discussed in the previous chapter are discussed. These are observed as four distinct types who show differential effects of their mothers' specific variations of mothering and care.

Basic theory about these infants' behaviors are described, as well as findings that define the groundwork for successful interventions for them based upon that theory. The theory and observations in chapters three and four are the groundwork. These set the stage for a broader understanding of and approach to parent and infant development in general.

The infants of the four types of severely emotionally disturbed mothers described in the previous chapter show differing effects of their mothers' distinct types of mothering and care, which will be described here.

TYPE 1 INFANTS: INFANTS OF THE SCHIZOPHRENIC MOTHER, PREDOMINANTLY NON-PARANOID TYPE

The Type 1 infant, a product of the Type 1 schizophrenic non-paranoid mothering, who lacks stimulation, will tend to accommodate to this and will become relatively non-responsive. For example, he/she will cease to seek eye contact (Fraiberg, 1980) and possibly to avoid eye contact (gaze aversion), and later on tend to avoid interpersonal contact with others. The Type 1 infant will tend not to be very alert, and will tend to lack motivation and curiosity. This Type 1 infant will tend to be underdeveloped physically, unless there are specific problems with overfeeding/eating. In general, the lack of stimulation will result increasingly in an infant who is small in size, unresponsive, and apathetic. Such infants tend to be underdeveloped in the cognitive area as well, may be developmentally delayed, and later may appear to have low intelligence (see Table 4.1).

TYPE 2 INFANTS: INFANTS OF PARANOID SCHIZOPHRENIC MOTHERING

The Type 2 infant, a product of the Type 2 paranoid schizophrenic mother, who is handled with intrusive overstimulation, will react to this in a typical manner. He/she will develop well physically and perhaps cognitively, because of the high level of stimulation. The infant will be highly attuned to the mother's expectation of him/her. (A constant, "pasted on" smile was observed in one such infant. This was in order to be acceptable and approved of by the mother.) The Type 2 infant will be highly conforming to mother's expectations since the mother's rigidity and stereotyped form of interactions do not allow for deviations. Free expression is not allowed, and experimentation in learning will be highly controlled by the mother. Consequently the infant's mood will not be a happy one, although a "forced" or required show of happiness may be observed. If the infant is not involved in the paranoid system of the mother, he/she may grow into a physically and intellectually well developed child. This is the case particularly if the mother is seen as "different/strange." Then the child may be able to make an adjustment to this. The child can separate him/herself from this strangeness and develop a separate identity. The child is then able to function well, though haunted by negative affect.

However, if the Type 2 infant is involved in the mother's paranoid system, the child will tend to develop much more severe problems. This is especially true if the child cannot separate him/herself from the mother.

Table 4.1
Negative Factors and Their Effects in the Schizophrenic Non-Paranoid Syndrome

Negative Factor	*Behavior*	*Mothering*	*The Infant*
Fear	Avoidance of contact with other people	Lack of holding baby ("log effect") Lack of eye contact Lack of auditory stimulation Lack of vestibular stimulation	Learns to expect little from other people Avoids others Gaze aversion Underdevelopment physically Poor alertness Lack of motivation and curiosity
Anxiety	Bizarre behavior Hallucinations Delusions	Unrealistic perceptions and expectations of the baby	Frustrated Feels incapable Afraid to try
Depression	Depressed behavior	Less interactive with baby Less responsive to baby's needs Less enthusiasm and interest in child	Feels rejected and incapable of pleasing others Incapable of self-determination Helplessness
Defenses	Obsessive-compulsive Phobic Sexual disturbances Gender identity Eating problems Substance abuse Dissociative problems	Rigid, stereotyped Overcontrolling Sexually abusive Neglect of the infant	Feels must conform May not explore Anxious about others Anxious in contact with the world Timid, seclusive High levels of fear and anxiety may result in symptom formation in the child

For instance, if in the mother's paranoid system the child is seen somehow as evil, the child may be physically or emotionally harmed. The infant may consequently be highly fearful and anxious. This will lead the child to develop his/her own psychopathology and strong defenses. Due to the very high level of stimulation and attention paid to the child, he/she may, at the same time, develop well in other realms, physically and intellectually (see Table 4.2).

Table 4.2
Negative Factors and Their Effects in Paranoid Schizophrenia

Negative Factor*	Behavior	Mothering	The Infant
Fear	Denial of fears Projections of fears and impulses	Intrusive behavior in holding, eye contact, auditory and vestibular stimulation, etc.	Highly sensitized to mother's expectations May develop well physically and intellectually
Anxiety	Denial of anxiety Projections of anxieties	Rigid, stereotyped interactions Freezing in behavior	Need to conform to expectations
Defenses	Paranoid ideation	Involving paranoid ideation (the in- fant is included within the para- noid framework)	The infant may be physically or emo- tionally harmed, depending upon specifics. The child may be highly fearful and anxious, and con- sequently develop its own severe psy- chopathology and strong defenses.
		Non-involving paranoid ideation (the infant is not included within the paranoid framework)	The child may come to recognize the mother's idio- syncratic ideation and consequently be able to learn to separate self from this. May be able to function well.

*Depression is not shown in this table because it is not necessarily inordinately present. Its presence will vary widely across mothers, and its consequent effects on mothering and the infant will vary accordingly.

TYPE 3 INFANTS: INFANTS OF BIPOLAR MOTHERING

The Type 3 infant, a product of the Type 3 bipolar mother, and who is interacted with non-contingently, will develop a sense of being unable to impact upon his/her environment. Since the infant's basic needs are met, though not upon the infant's demands, he/she will learn to wait passively. The infant will feel helpless to effect the satisfaction of its needs, and a sense of helplessness will predominate. The only thing the infant can do is wait and watch what will happen. The child will therefore be alert and vigilant to the world around it. In general the Type 3 child will be passive, alert, vigilant, and have a sense of helplessness (see Table 4.3).

As this Type 3 infant develops language (thought) and then begins to ask "why?" about the world, he/she will also ask why he/she is unable to have an effect upon the mother. The inevitable answer is that it must be "because I am not worthwhile." The child thus develops a sense of worthlessness (Gochman, 1985; Weary and Mirel, 1982). The sense of worthlessness, once well ingrained, tends to be intractable. No evidence encountered in life is able to be accepted to contradict the basic sense of worthlessness; all positives can be rationalized away. The sense of helplessness and worthlessness set the foundation for a depressive syndrome.

Table 4.3
Negative Factors and Their Effects in Bipolar Disorders

*Negative Factors**	*Behavior*	*Mothering*	*The Infant*
Depression	Varies between depressed and manic	Non-contingent interactions	Passive
	Preoccupation with self-enhancement		Alert
	Lack of intrinsic interest in others		Vigilant
			Helpless
			With the development of language, the child will start to develop the *anlage* for a depressive syndrome.

*The other three factors—fear, anxiety, and defenses—are not shown in this table because here they are not necessarily inordinately present. Though they may be present, they will vary widely, and their consequent effects on mothering and the infant will vary accordingly.

Table 4.4
Negative Factors and Their Effects in Major Depression

Negative Factors*	Behavior	Mothering	The Infant
Depression	Diminished activity level	Diminished interactions	Passive
	Preoccupation with depressive thoughts		Later may develop toward self-sufficiency early in life
	Interest in others—hoping not to be rejected; avoid behavior that might result in rejection		

*The other three factors—fear, anxiety, and defenses—are not shown in this table because here they are not necessarily inordinately present. Though they may be present, they will vary widely, and their consequent effects on mothering and the infant will vary accordingly.

TYPE 4 INFANTS: INFANTS OF MAJOR DEPRESSION-MOTHERING

The Type 4 mother, who is suffering from a major depression, tends not to be able to care for her infant. Overall, mother-infant interactions are diminished. When she is able to garner some energy, she will show interest in the child but will interact minimally. The Type 4 infant tends to make an adjustment to this and to become passive (see Table 4.4).

The mother will try to meet the infant's needs. As he/she grows, the Type 4 child may of necessity become relatively self-sufficient early on. Much depends upon other influences in the child's life—the family and other social systems. Furthermore, the mother's depression frequently abates to some extent, in which case she will tend to become more active with the child. The interaction will then vary across cases according to the degree of depression and other psychodynamics.

CONCLUSION

The negative factors of fear, anxiety, and depression, as well as typical defenses, when examined in relation to four types of severely emotionally disturbed, psychotic mothers, show typical resultant behaviors, mothering styles, and effects on the infants. These findings serve to provide a conceptual framework with which to observe mother and infant interactions and to provide understanding. The findings provide a basis upon which to build a framework of specific and appropriate interventions.

SOME QUESTIONS AND ANSWERS

In the Type 1 schizophrenic non-paranoid mother, what is the effect of fear on her behavior?

Fear will create a general avoidance behavior in the Type 1 non-paranoid mother. She will tend to avoid contact with other people in general, and she will have specific avoidance behavior, such as avoidance of eye contact, of touching others, and of getting involved in an integrated manner with others. This kind of behavior will also be present in relation to her child, where it will tend to express itself in the lack of eye contact with the baby and in generally not stimulating the baby in many ways. There will be little in the way of holding or cuddling the baby, of baby talk or singing to the baby, moving or rocking it, and so on. The overall effect will be a dearth of stimulation of her child. The effect of this type of mothering on the infant will be a dampening one. The infant attempts, from the earliest age, to try to make eye contact. When the experience is that the mother avoids it, and that he/she is unable to make eye contact with the mother, there will be a giving up on that score. Furthermore, if the infant is not held in a gently molding fashion, the baby will learn not to expect to be comforted. In its frustration, the baby will start to avoid eye contact and will display gaze aversion, turning its head away from the mother. Because of the lack of adequate stimulation, the infant will develop poor alertness. That is, since nothing is expected to be forthcoming, he/she will not be alert to stimulation.

Lack of relatedness between the mother and the infant, due to this kind of handling, will interfere with the attachment process between the two. The general level of motivation and curiosity will also be negatively affected, and the child will evidence lacks in those areas. Eventually, barring other influences, as it grows, the child will learn to expect little from other people, may tend to be physically underdeveloped, and will in turn tend to avoid contact with others.

What is the effect of anxiety on the Type 1 schizophrenic non-paranoid mother?

The effect of anxiety is a disorganization of behavior and perception. The Type 1 mother will consequently tend to display some bizarre behaviors and may well have delusions, which are distortions in thinking. If the disorder is severe, she may also have hallucinations, which is a disorder in perception. In terms of behavior vis-à-vis the child, the Type 1 mother's anxiety will foster her unrealistic expectations of the baby. Her needs are so great, and her distortions so heightened by the anxiety, that she tends not to be able to see the baby for what it is. The newborn child does not have speech or perceptions, cannot think or have motivations, does not attribute feelings or motivations to the mother. The mother's perceptions will tend to reflect her own needs, unrealistically disregarding the nature and abilities of the baby. For instance, the mother may expect to obtain emotional support from a one-month-old baby. This is completely unrealistic. When the baby then fails to be sensitive to the needs of the mother, and instead of giving her the support she wants, starts to cry and express its own needs, the mother will feel frustrated. She may see the baby as being "wise," or outsmarting her, or as being more mature in holding the bottle when it is too young to do so. She may misinterpret movements of the baby as being symbolic, when they are simply natural movements. Or she may see anger in the baby's eyes. The baby in turn will react to these unrealistic perceptions, expectations, and behaviors in developing a confusion as to what to expect, and consequently developing a feeling of being an incapable child because it cannot meet the needs of the mother. There will likely be a good deal of frustration on the part of the child. In fact, the child may develop the tendency to be afraid to try anything new because there is no certainty as to the reaction he/she is likely to receive from the mother.

What is the effect of depression on the Type 1 non-paranoid mother?

The depressed mother exhibits behavior that is less active and less reactive. The extent of the lessening of the activity and reactivity levels will depend upon the degree of her depression. As a result she will be less responsive to her baby. She will tend to interact much less spontaneously with the baby, so that there will be less, or no, playful interchange with it. There will be a lessening of touching, rocking, cuddling, and verbal interaction with the baby. The amount of baby talk, talking and singing to the baby, will be lessened, and perhaps absent if the depression is severe enough. The depression will also tend to lessen the degree of responsiveness of the mother to the baby's needs. For instance, if the baby cries because of hunger, the tendency to respond to that cry by giving a bottle/feeding the baby will be lessened. In extreme depression, this may affect the mother to be essentially non-responsive to the needs of the baby. The mother's total interest in and enthusiasm for the child will be dampened to the extent that there is depression present in this mother. Affective reactivity to the baby will also be lessened. The baby, in turn, will experience this as rejection by the mother. The child will try to please the mother but, because of her general lack of reactivity, will not receive reactions from the mother in his/her attempts to please her. The baby will develop the feeling that he/she is incapable of pleasing others. Since the mother tends not to respond to the demands of the baby to have its needs met, it will, over time, develop the feeling that it is incapable of self-determination, that is, of affecting others to have its needs met. The feeling is then also translated into a sense of helplessness on the part of the baby.

What is the effect of defenses on the Type 1 non-paranoid mother?

Defenses can take many forms. The person may have developed defenses that are of an obsessive-compulsive nature. In that case the behavior would reflect a meticulousness in the person's repeating acts. The typical example of checking and rechecking that the gas is off is a minor, simple example. Once an idea is developed, the person may obsessively ruminate about it, not being able to rid him/herself of it. Or she may need to follow a certain ritual compulsively before eating, or before taking a step in any direction, or in the process of performing any task. These are self-absorbing and very rigid types of behavior, which are typical of obsessive compulsive symptomatology. The obsessive-compulsive symptom will tend to create a rigid stereotyped interaction in mothering. The mother will tend to be unbending. She will tend to be inflexible in her responses to the baby, regardless of the baby's needs. The obsessive-compulsive symptomatology also tends to create an overcontrolling type of behavior toward the baby. The rigidity and overcontrolling qualities are stultifying to the child. For instance, in trying to teach a child how to write, a mother may put her hand on top of the child's or push the child's hand to form the letters. An occasional behavior of this kind may not be noxious. However, when this is part of an obsessive-compulsive pattern, and is the typical interaction pattern, which is highly confining and frustrating, it creates a feeling within the child that he/she must conform to the mother and is not allowed to explore different ways of doing things or different things to do, but must do exactly what the mother wants. Other kinds of defenses may include, for instance, phobic reactions on the part of the mother. She may be phobic in relation to many types of situations, such as the dark, heights, and so on. This will constrict her general functioning. It will tend to make for a tense kind of mothering behavior. The baby will tend to react in an anxious way to the tension felt in the mother. Defenses may also be sexual disturbances, eating problems, substance abuse problems, dissociative problems, for example, which will cause resultant behaviors in the mother. These might include sexual abuse of the child, overfeeding or underfeeding the child, or neglect of the child. Because of the general preoccupation of the mother with her own symptomatology, and because of the specific impact of her psychopathology, the infant will grow to be anxious in his/her contact with the world, timid and seclusive, and tend to regard others with caution. The child will start to form symptoms of his/her own in reaction to these fears and anxieties. Just as the defenses of the mother can vary widely, the consequent reactions in the infant will also have a wide range.

How is it that the Type 2 paranoid schizophrenic mother intrusively overstimulates the baby?

To the extent that the Type 2 mother is well defended she will be assertive about her property, needs, and ideas. Since her baby is seen as hers, she will tend to show her interest in her child by asserting her property rights in relation to him/her. In her rigidity she will tend to express this consistently. She will do what she wants to do with her baby. Basically, beneath the defenses, the same dynamic structures are present as in the Type 1 non-paranoid schizophrenic. There will be a fear of the baby. However, the fear is handled through denial. This expresses itself in her behavior with the baby, for instance, in doing a great deal of grooming, such as combing his/her hair, cleaning the fingernails, and picking at the ears and eyes to clean them. The problem with this is that it is a persistent behavior. She will at the same time tend to lack empathic interaction with the baby. Her interaction will not be consistent with the needs of her baby. In small doses, the stimulation the mother provides may appear positive. Observed over a period of twenty minutes or longer, it will be clear that it is overly rigid and unrelenting. In sum, it is noxious stimulation.

Why is it an advantage to the child to see the Type 2 paranoid schizophrenic mother as "different" or strange?

The child is intruded upon and made to feel highly controlled in a non-empathic fashion. There are compelling behaviors on the part of the mother in relation to the child, which are typically outside of the norm, making demands on the child which could be extremely disturbing and anxiety arousing. This is particularly the case if the child is very much confused and consequently feels even more controlled by the mother. If the child is able to see her as a strange person, that means that the child has been able to see the reality of the mother and separate him/herself from that bizarre reality, resulting in less confusion. The ability to separate from the mother in this way is much more likely if the mother has not included the child in her delusional system. It is much more difficult if the child is part of her delusions. For instance, if the mother's delusion requires her to see the child as a devil, and consequently send the child into the basement for long periods of time, the child will suffer very directly from this delusion, and since the mother attributes particular noxious characteristics to the child within the delusional system, the child will have difficulties in separating his/her own thinking from the mother's. For example, if she consistently treats the child as bad, and uses extreme measures to deal with this, the natural reaction of the child will be to buy into that process by attributing to itself the characteristic of being bad.

How does the Type 2 paranoid schizophrenic mother's lack of empathy for the child express itself?

The mother's needs are extremely pressing. She has strong fears and anxieties. This is a basic assumption in that she has developed the tightest defensive system available in the paranoid ideation. She is highly defended. However, her strong needs are the forces that propel her. She will, in interacting with the baby, attempt to meet her own needs. There is very little energy left on her part to deal with the needs of the baby, because she has mobilized her energies to such a high extent to defend herself from her anxieties and fears. When she talks to the baby, it is for her own gratification. When she plays with the baby, it is for her own gratification. When she tries to teach the child to make a circle on paper, for instance, she may tend to demand that that circle be perfect in front of the therapist. (In that instance the mother's motivation was to impress the therapist through the child, as an extension of herself.) An example is the mother who, for the first seven months of the baby's life, played with her incessantly and never let anyone else take care of the baby in any way. She suddenly proclaimed that she was gong to work full time. She said she would let her mother take care of the baby. The inconsistency demonstrates that her motivation was not for the baby's sake, but rather had to do with her own needs. She played with the baby to entertain herself and meet other personal needs. These were easily supplanted in a manner irrelevant to the baby, in her abruptly giving up essentially the complete care of the baby, without any concern for the child. She did not question how the child would react or feel about this abrupt change. A more bizarre example is the mother who took care of her baby for three months. When this became too burdensome for her, she developed a delusion which propelled her to go to the butcher requesting that he chop up the baby.

What is the effect of fear on the Type 2 paranoid schizophrenic mother?

The paranoid reactions to negative feelings or emotions of any kind are attempts to deny and repress these. Consequently there will be a denial of fears. However, they will tend to surface in projections of those fears and impulses onto other people. If the denial is functioning well, the person is then free to express his/her assertiveness in attempts to meet his/her own needs. The assertiveness may be expressed in mothering behavior. What is typically seen is intrusiveness in the mother's interaction with the baby, usually in many or all modalities of stimulation. The mother may pick at the baby in excessive grooming or talk a great deal to the baby. Because of the unrelenting nature and lack of sensitivity to the needs of the child, the behavior tends to be experienced as intrusive and annoying. The baby cannot escape the mother. The infant tends to become highly sensitized to the mother's expectations and tries to conform to them. At the same time, the mother tends to stimulate the baby a great deal. Though this may be noxious, it is nevertheless stimulation. The baby will tend to grow well physically and intellectually, unless there are extenuating circumstances.

What is the effect of anxiety on the Type 2 paranoid schizophrenic mother?

Denial is the major reaction to the anxiety. If the denial is effective, it will reduce the anxiety sizably. There may be projections onto other people. Behavior tends to be locked into rigid, stereotyped patterns. The enormous degree of denial used to deal with the anxiety will not allow for fluidity and flexibility in the mother's interactions with her baby. She will tend to impose rigid standards on the baby and not be open to the child's or anyone else's ideas, nor be open to reciprocity and negotiation. In other words, she will insist that things have to be done the way she wants them. The child will react by developing a need to conform to the mother's expectations. Conformity then becomes a generalized pattern for the child.

What is the effect of defenses on the Type 2 paranoid schizophrenic mother?

The prime defense that is utilized by the paranoid schizophrenic mother is paranoid type ideation. There are systematized delusions with which she is preoccupied. She may have auditory hallucinations, which are in all likelihood tied to the delusional system. The person's behavior may follow from the ideas that she has in her delusion. Depending on the strength of the delusion, she will tend to act on it to a greater or lesser extent. In terms of mothering behavior, the delusions break down into two basic categories. The mother may maintain the delusional system she had prior to the advent of the child, and not include the child in her delusional ideation. These would be non-involving delusions. On the other hand, she may include the infant within the paranoid framework. The delusions would, in that case, include/involve the baby. This is a much more at-risk situation for the baby. If the delusion, for instance, is that the baby is potentially harmful, bad, or evil, then the mother may act within that framework, against him/her and be emotionally or physically harmful to the baby, depending on the specific content of the ideas that she has about the child. The child, having experienced harmful acts, will become fearful and anxious in relation to the mother. On a continuing basis, the child will tend to develop his/her own psychopathology. However, if the paranoid ideation does not involve the infant, and the mother continues with her paranoid delusions, as the child grows up, the child may tend to notice the strangeness of the mother. The child will be able to see it as strange because he/she is not being put directly at risk by the mother. If the child is able to separate him/herself, to recognize that the mother has strange ideas, which are not related to him/herself, he/she will be much less affected or harmed by the mother's delusional system. The child may, as a consequence, be able to develop into a well-functioning adult. However, the burden of having to deal with a mother who is so strange will leave its effect upon the person. Typically these children, though they may escape severe psychopathology and may develop well intellectually, will always tend to feel burdened and be sad about the mother's situation.

How is it that the bipolar mother interacts in a non-contingent manner with her baby?

The bipolar mother's core problem is a sense of worthlessness. She is driven by this sense of worthlessness to attempt, in whatever manner possible, to gain some sense of worth. She will, in all her actions, have self-enhancement as her central motivation. That is, if she studies, it will be in order to hear other people say that she is a good student. The intrinsic learning of the material she studies will not be the prime issue. If she interacts with other people, then her central motivation will be to have them think of her as wonderful, smart, powerful, and so on. The intrinsic interaction will not be her primary interest. Unfortunately, since the sense of worthlessness is a basic assumption, it will not be conducive to change as a result of evidence to the contrary. For instance, if she does very well in her studies, this will tend to be rationalized and not be taken as a true enhancement of her sense of worth. Though that is the objective, it will tend not to succeed. It is an extremely intransigent assumption which drives this mother. In relation to the baby, she will similarly act to try to enhance her sense of worth. The specifics of this action will depend on what behaviors she values in child care. If she feels that being a good mother is important, as most women do, her behavior with the baby will have as the basic motivation that other people think she is a good mother. In other words, she will try to enhance her self-image. Since the basic motivation is self-enhancement, it typically does not require contingent interactions with the child. Her preoccupation will divert her attention from the needs of the child. If she is not too severely manic or depressive at that time, she will take care of the child and meet its basic needs, but in a non-contingent fashion. The mother will tend to feed the baby when it is convenient for her, or when she happens to think of it, or when someone else is present whose opinion she values. She will not tend to react to the baby in terms of the baby's momentary needs. The child may cry for hunger, but remains unfed. If this continues over time, he/she will learn that feeding does not occur in response to crying but is unpredictable. The child will learn not to cry because his/her demands do not achieve results, but rather to become vigilant, watching and listening carefully for signs of impending gratification. The major problem for the child is that this pattern creates passivity and a sense of helplessness. This manner of interaction is typical for the mother whether she is in a relatively manic or depressive state or in remission. The basic dynamics remain the same, though the behavior changes. If the mother becomes too depressed or too manic, she may not take care of the baby during that time.

How is it that the child attributes the reason for the mother's non-contingent interactions to him/herself?

The mother's acting in terms of her needs for self-enhancement tends to look like random behavior. Sometimes when the baby cries, she feeds it, sometimes not. Sometimes it is shortly thereafter; sometimes it takes longer. There is no consistency, and therefore a lack of relatedness, between the child's crying and having that need met. The experienced perception is that this is random behavior. The child tries to understand why this random behavior is encountered. It is a puzzle. Since the child, at the time of language development, is also at an egocentric stage, he/she will tend to attribute events to him/herself. When he/she asks the question "Why is it that I cannot have an effect on my mother's actions?", the child tends to relate the answer to him/herself: "It must be something about me that makes my mother not react to me." Since it is experienced as a rejection, "it must be that there is something about me that is to be rejected." This means that "I am not worthwhile."

Is there a circularity in this process?
Yes. The mother who feels worthless treats the child in such a way that the child starts to assume that he/she is worthless.

What is the fundamental dynamic difference between bipolar depression and major depression?
The basic dynamic in bipolar depression is that the person is trying to enhance him/herself in order to feel less worthless, whereas in major depression the person is driven by guilt feelings.

When the mother with major depression is somewhat less depressed, so that she is able to care for her child, what is the major effect of that depression?
The depression will tend directly to diminish her activity level. She will tend to be less reactive to the child in that she will not be able to garner her energies to interact with it. Beyond that, due to the guilt feelings that permeate the major depressive, she will generally have an interest in other people, hoping that they not reject her. When she is feeling vulnerable, she will avoid others in order to protect herself from possible rejection. This includes her interaction with the baby, where interaction will also be diminished in order to protect herself. She wants very much to be accepted by the baby, but will tend to be afraid of possible rejection. Major depression does tend to lift with time. The baby will, however, have learned to be passive because of the insecurity engendered by the lack of interaction by the mother. If the somewhat older child has had to take care of him/herself, and perhaps has even had to help in the care of the mother, then it may be that this child will develop competencies early and become relatively more self-sufficient. This will be at the sacrifice of the freedom most children have during the formative years to play and explore. There will tend to be a dampening of the spirit in this child.

5

Basic Principles and Techniques
of Dyadic Psychotherapy

Before examining in greater detail what occurs when dyadic psychotherapy interventions are applied to infants and parents, based upon the theoretical concepts outlined in chapters 3 and 4, we will look at some principles, techniques, and types of interventions utilized in infant/parent psychotherapy.

This chapter sets out some general basic principles and techniques of dyadic psychotherapy that may be used with any population ranging from the severely disturbed psychotic mother to the "normal" mother. In any dyadic psychotherapy process, assessment is primary. The elements of what to look for in the evaluation of the infant and in the evaluation of the parent are noted.

The author reports the specific differences in her findings on a diagnostic spectrum between discrete patterns of specific interventions with the severely disturbed parent. This is followed by a general discussion of the dyadic psychotherapy process and the role of the beginning psychotherapist in learning and utilizing dyadic psychotherapy.

Some do's and don'ts of dyadic psychotherapy are also given, in order to clarify the general methodology of this work with infants and parents based upon my research findings and clinical work.

Dyadic psychotherapy is a psychotherapeutic intervention that has been developed specifically for mother and child (Gochman, 1986). It is an attempt to intervene in the developmental relationship as it emerges and develops between mother and infant. Therefore, once the infant is born, the therapeutic intervention program of dyadic psychotherapy is planned to encompass the infant as well as the mother. The father and significant others will also be included, when they are available.

ASSESSMENTS

One always begins with evaluations of infant functioning, behavior, and adaptive potentials. An assessment also is done of the mother's strengths and weaknesses in her ability to interact with her infant in a positive reciprocal fashion. Her ability to relate to significant others and to deal with her reality situation are likewise assessed.

What To Look for in Dyadic Psychotherapy Assessments

Assessments may include the use of conventional clinical assessment modalities, which include infant testing. The assessment always includes observations of the mother and infant dyad interaction in an unstructured, free situation. Such observation allows for an assessment of the degree and quality of the interaction. It includes an assessment of the interaction in the various sensory modalities: vestibular, auditory, visual, and tactile. It is significant to observe the molding between mother and infant, the eye contact, the rocking/moving-soothing of the baby, the baby talk/singing-cooing, the petting, and touching. The amount of these behaviors is observed, in order to assess whether enough or too much stimulation is taking place, as well as to determine the quality of the interactions. Actions are observed to note the soothing, intrusive, contingent, or non-contingent quality of the behavior.

With seriously disturbed or psychotic mothers, there are specific issues for the therapist to focus on. Differences in the dyadic interaction exist on a diagnostic basis. Non-paranoid schizophrenic mothers under-stimulate their infants. On the other hand, paranoid schizophrenic mothers tend to overstimulate, intrusively. Bipolar mothers are typified by non-contingent interactions. There are, of course, variations dependent upon the degree of psychopathology in the mother and the degree of anxiety and depression.

Treatment plans are based on the above, plus the type and amount of support the mother has in the family and community (see Appendix). Appropriate agencies are contacted and involved in a coordinated manner as clinically indicated. These can be quite numerous and the process complex, perhaps requiring separate case management.

Disturbances in Childrearing

When the mother is severely disturbed, there tend to be profound interferences with childrearing. Four types of patterns have been noted.

One type is the mother who is extremely frightened in her mothering role. She is afraid that she will harm the baby and consequently is closed off from interacting. This causes a dearth of stimulation and an inability to attain joy in the relationship. It is a highly constricted relationship. One mother, Liz, typically sat with her baby across her lap, not looking at, touching, talking to, or moving (rocking) the baby. She was afraid of other people, did not look into their eyes when talking with them, and did the same with her little baby. Though Liz did have concerns and feelings about her, this was not evident in her interactions with her child. The baby, in turn, became passive and stopped initiating interactions with her mother. Liz thought that the baby's moving her arms was dangerous (a bizarre thought) and said that she needed to be walked around the block when she stretched (to keep bad things from happening to her). Such bizarre interactions and ideation further complicate the picture.

The second interactional pattern occurs when the mother egocentrically overidentifies with the baby. In this case, a symbiotic relationship develops in which the mother overstimulates the baby, making constant demands on it. As a result, the baby becomes extremely alert and responsive but very much overburdened with the constant responsibility of meeting the mother's demands. One mother, Beatrice, was so implicitly demanding that the baby smiled constantly. When she awoke, before opening her eyes, a smile formed. The smile was ever present, except on rare occasions when Beatrice was not interacting with her. The child was at risk for severe rejection and punishment should she deviate in the slightest from the mother's wishes and expectations.

The third pattern is typified by non-contingent interaction. In this case, the mother's basic dynamic is one of feeling worthless and helpless, which tends to result in extreme depression. Attempts at compensation result in hypomania. When this cycle exhausts itself, there is a return to the basic depression. The patient in this instance is preoccupied with ego-enhancement. She experiences everything in terms of herself, searching to bolster her meager feelings of worth. In mothering she wants only to be "a good mother." She wants to be seen by others as showing concern and interest, and as doing what a good mother should do. She will consequently care for the child in terms of how she thinks others will perceive her. However, she will be insensitive to the child's needs. That is, her own needs to bolster her feelings of worth supersede all. The interactions with the baby are typified by a lack of contingency. The baby's cries may be ignored. Feeding takes place at the mother's convenience and in a manner that suits the mother rather than taking the baby into account. The infant experiences a powerlessness; he/she cannot influence the mother's caring behavior. The infant therefore, in turn, develops a sense of helplessness and later develops a feeling of basic worthlessness, thereby perpetuating the mother's own dynamics.

A fourth pattern found is typified by diminished interactions. In this case, the mother's basic dynamic is dominated by guilt feelings and fear of rejection, with massive depression. The mother consequently is hesitant to reach out to the baby. She makes an effort not to alienate the child. Although she is aware of the needs of the child, she has little psychic energy to try to meet these needs. The degree of interaction with her infant will vary with the depth of the depression. The infant will tend to adjust by becoming passive.

These are the discrete patterns found in work done with an extremely disturbed population. There are, of course, a myriad of other patterns of pathological mother-child interactions found at all levels.

Many patterns of interaction are based on a lack of emotional skills on the part of the mother, whether disturbed or "normal," to interact advantageously with her child. The building blocks for the development of coping abilities and for emotional security will consequently be faulty. Emotional problems on the part of the parents place the child at risk. Immaturity, at one end of the continuum, and older motherhood at the other may create problems. Sensory or motor disabilities in the child, or similar disabilities in the parents, may also create at-risk situations.

THE DYADIC PSYCHOTHERAPY PROCESS

The first step in therapeutic intervention is, as always, the establishment of a *therapeutic alliance*. It is a key process issue for the very disturbed mother to experience the therapist as competent to deal with her extremely strong fears and impulses. The dyadic parent-infant therapist, in general, needs to be seen by the mother as an understanding person who is capable of dealing with the therapeutic situation. The severely disturbed mother is particularly open to, and in need of, the supportive approach in the therapeutic relationship. The mother with a young child offers a special opportunity for the therapist to use supportive interventions.

Another advantageous intervention with severely disturbed mothers is the use of *demystification*. The objective in demystification is to cut through the most frightening aspect of the problem, using reality, in order to reduce the anxiety and allow the patient to feel in control of her own reactions. For instance, in the psychotic patient, an explanation of the nature of hallucinations is very much in order. For example, a young woman heard voices of her "earth angels" telling her that she was all right. This first occurred when she was six years old after she had been sexually abused. Her family situation offered her no emotional support, and she saw herself all alone in a hostile world. It was disorganizing to her to hear voices when she knew deep down that they were not real. Though soothing, hearing the voices made her feel "crazy." This created additional tension and fear, and excacerbated her confused thinking, thereby also increasing her anxiety. The use of demystification was very much in order. When discussing the original experience which occurred at age six, the therapist said "you so much needed a guardian angel to protect you, you imagined it so strongly in your tremendous loneliness, fear, and need, and then you heard the voices." There was tremendous relief at this demystification (which at the same time did not remove the legitimacy of the voices, which were her only support). The "crazy" feeling about herself lifted, and she was able to proceed productively in her therapy.

There are similarities of dyadic psychotherapy to other forms of psychotherapy. For example, a variety of psychotherapeutic approaches are utilized, including supportive interpretations and psychodynamic interpretations; interpretation of the dynamics of mother-infant interactions; interpretations of the mother's transference to the baby; translation to the mother of infant behavior so as to indicate the child's needs. In early-involving psychosis, in which the child is seen as the persecutor of the mother, maneuvers to avoid and to disassociate such ideas in relation to the infant are also used. Further techniques are used, such as modeling, behavioral directives, suggestions, infant stimulation techniques, and psychoeducational techniques, as appropriate to the situation.

It is important for the dyadic therapist to know the mother's personal history and to understand her psychodynamic functioning. This can help the therapist empathically to trigger the mother's emotional responses by drawing from the client's past experience and/or from transference. For example, if the therapist knows of an experience in which the mother felt rejected, he/she can remind the mother of that feeling and its context. Thus the mother's empathy for the infant is fostered. For example, after having been ignored by her mother for some minutes, a toddler stood staring into space, now not paying attention to her mother's attempt to engage her in play. The mother, Tricia, was feeling hurt and started to withdraw. Tricia had suffered in feeling the "outsider" who was brought up by an aunt together with her own children. Tricia was also sickly as a child, and the aunt would send her to her room to "rest." She did not want to spend time in her room; she had wanted to play with the other children. This had always created a feeling of rejection in Tricia. In the present therapeutic moment, Tricia showed no evidence of empathy for her toddler. The germinal phases of a negative interplay were at hand. The therapist said (speaking for the toddler): "Oh mommy! I feel so left out!" then: "just as you used to feel when you had to stay in your room." This brought forth an immediate empathic response from Tricia; she stroked the toddler's head and tried again to engage her.

The therapist should also convey an appreciation of and understanding for the intrapsychic struggles of the mother. The mother struggles between meeting the needs of her infant and her own strong needs, as well as with her frequently distorted perceptions. The therapist should conduct therapy with sensitivity to the courage and immensity of the mother's task.

There are also significant differences between dyadic psychotherapy and other psychotherapies. Perhaps the most comprehensive way of characterizing the differences from conventional therapy is to point out that the intervention in parent/infant dyadic psychotherapy is within an in-vivo process of development, as demonstrated in the here-and-now of the psychotherapy sessions. That is, although at times there may be some retrospective work, the bulk of therapeutic intervention is going to be aimed at the momentary happenings within the session and within the dyad. We are dealing with the developmental process of both the relationship between the mother and child and of the child itself. The therapist's task in this form of psychotherapy is doubly complex. The therapist simultaneously needs to maintain both an active, often vivacious, interrelationship with the mother and also with the infant. However, the therapist needs to avoid indicating a superiority of mothering skills, at the same time maintaining a stance of expertise. The therapist needs to balance between the passive and the active role. That is, to be sufficiently active to express interest and enthusiasm for the growing relationship and for the growing baby, while at the same time consistently reinforcing the mother's role and the mother's importance in the therapy situation.

The practiced conventional psychotherapist tends to have difficulty in abandoning the more conventional role of maintaining a passive, neutral, reflective nature, and shifting to a much more active and interactive psychodynamic stance. The conventional therapist role has to be abandoned in order to participate as described above. One mechanism that is helpful to the beginning dyadic psychotherapist has been conceptualized. It is to ask the therapist to think of him/herself in the place of the baby, and then to conceptualize the baby's experiences and try to express and interpret them to the mother in the here-and-now situation. This has been found to be a helpful aid in guiding a new therapist into assuming the dyadic psychotherapy model. At the same time, great care must be taken to maintain constant empathy with the mother and to make interpretations in her terms.

The basic attempt is: (1) to involve the mother in a therapeutic alliance; (2) to maintain an ongoing involvement of the mother with the infant; (3) to reinforce all nurturing acts and behaviors on the mother's part; and (4) to try to supplement these behaviors through other therapeutic means. For example, when the mother does not exhibit a specific behavior important to the infant, the therapist may set out to model this behavior. It is important to execute this modeling in a sensitive manner, so that the mother is never made to feel that she is not doing an adequate job. Her mothering role is never usurped. The baby is not held or taken by the therapist unless, and until, there is expressed permission by the mother to do so. This is to help the mother feel that she is not being threatened in any way by the therapist's establishing a relationship with the infant to her exclusion.

In the case of the schizophrenic mother, even more so than others, there is a tendency to identify very strongly with the new baby. The newness of the situation, the identification with the baby, and the desire to do well in her relationship with the baby tend to provide a motivation that is peculiar and strong at this time in the schizophrenic woman's life. It, therefore, appears to be an advantageous time for the therapeutic intervention. The mother wants very much to be able to take care of her baby adequately. However, she typically sees herself as unable to do so or is afraid of her inadequacy in mothering.

The non-paranoid mother also needs a great deal of support and encouragement to increase her stimulation of the infant, with whom she is afraid to interact. Often present is psychotic ideation about the baby, which needs to be clarified and interpreted in order to prevent these thoughts from being acted upon. For example, at the time her baby was one month old, Agnes, a schizophrenic mother, looked down at the baby and said, "His eyes are turning up just like mine" (this was a side effect of the prolixin she was taking). This was explored immediately. Agnes felt it was an indication that the baby would be psychotic when he grew up. In fact, the baby's eyes were not turning up but simply moving naturally. Her thinking was clarified in the therapy process, and the thought of the baby's psychotic development did not reappear.

The paranoid schizophrenic mother tends to stimulate the baby a great deal, unless she is concomitantly very much depressed. The problematic aspects of mothering tend to center around the delusional system. It is particularly dangerous if the mother includes the baby in her delusions. An example is a paranoid schizophrenic mother, Rose, who, under stress, started to see her baby as one of her persecutors. Her voices told Rose to take the baby to the zoo and feed it to the lions. In this type of situation, it is urgent for the therapist to intervene and to interpret and clarify, in trying to disinvolve the child. Furthermore, the paranoid schizophrenic mother tends toward a tight symbiotic development. The danger to the child is in having to walk a tightrope of pleasing the mother. This needs to be looked at therapeutically and clarified. It is, of course, always important to deal with the mother on her terms, at her level, about her concerns and in her interest.

The bipolar patient offers a different picture (Gochman, 1985). For this type of patient the feeling of worthlessness is at the core. She consequently has little psychic energy left for the child on its own terms. However, the child, perceived as a vehicle for self-enhancement, is very important to her. This mother does not offer a stable base for the child. Although she may meet the child's basic needs, she is not dependable in meeting the child's demands. The child is therefore at risk for developing a sense of helplessness and passivity. The therapist can deal with the basic dynamics of the mother accordingly. It is unlikely that significant changes can be effected quickly enough in the mother to be of service to her present infant, who is developing rapidly. The mother will, however, attempt to perform for the therapist in order to try to enhance herself. This critical motive can be utilized to help attain mothering behaviors. However, any small slights to the mother's sense of worth, coming from any contacts in her daily life, can set a depressive or manic reaction into motion. Therefore, the presence of support people is typically essential. It may be that the father of the child can sustain the nurturing care needed. It may be that another relative needs to take on an active part. However, such families are frequently very much alone, having previously alienated all those around them. In that case, more formal support systems may need to be called upon, such as government or volunteer agencies. It is well for the therapist to anticipate this beforehand, in order to prepare the way for others to play a caregiving role.

The patient with a major depression is found to differ from the bipolar in having a somewhat higher level of ego strength, and so being able to tolerate their severe depression to a greater extent. The depression is often a reaction to a life event. When profoundly depressed, this mother is not capable of caring for her child, and help with child care is necessary. In the therapy process, the mother can be encouraged to explore her feelings which are at the core of her reticence to interact with her baby. She is encouraged to express her positive feelings in her interactions with her baby and to verbalize to the therapist concerning her negative feelings. As the mother starts to demonstrate her positive feelings, remarkably the infant reacts positively. The dyad is thereby gradually guided toward the development of a positive attachment. The attachment process also helps the mother abandon her depression by beginning to feel increasingly adequate in her mothering role, and it helps the infant in freeing him/her to develop on course.

SOME GENERAL DO'S AND DON'TS OF DYADIC PSYCHOTHERAPY

The Do's

Based on the author's findings, when working with a severely emotionally disturbed mother, the therapist needs to keep certain fundamental concepts in mind: the mother's basic psychodynamics; her available resources and support people; her intelligence level; her skills and abilities; her motivations in life; her general energy level (any illnesses that may affect this); whether or not she is taking any psychotropic medications and how these medications may affect her ability to function; the degree to which she is alone or has social contacts; her living/housing situation; whether or not she has the necessities of life such as food; her anxiety and depression levels and her symptoms; the degree of control she has, particularly in relation to her aggressive impulses; the effect significant others in her life have upon her; her ability to take care of her own basic needs and those of her infant; her concept of the mothering role; her concept of her infant and her feelings about him/her; and her ability to utilize professionals versus opposition toward them.

Regarding the infant, certain basics also need to be kept in mind: an undestanding of the infant; an understanding of the infant's adjustment to the caretaker; knowledge of any injuries, debilities, or illnesses; the condition at birth; the level of the baby's developmental functioning; the baby's temperament; and the impact that the baby has upon the mother and upon other adults in terms of cuteness and likeability, for example.

The Don'ts

When working with a severely emotionally disturbed mother, the following are generally counterindicated: using behavioral directives as the treatment modality of choice in most interventions; communicating to the mother that she is poor at mothering and that the therapist is better at it;

taking over the mothering functions by playing with the baby and caring for him (feeding, dressing, changing, and so on); being judgmental; sympathizing with the infant as opposed to the mother; allowing the mother to hurt/harm the infant during a session; listening to verbal material brought to the session that reflects having put the baby at risk or having the impulse to do so, without therapeutically intervening; neglecting the mother's needs for nurturance; being intrinsically dishonest with the mother in communicating a falsehood to her, such as saying that she is a good mother when this is not the therapist's opinion; or burdening her with a value of the therapist or of the society that the mother is not capable of fulfilling, and that would be destructive to the child (such as a "good" mother raises her own child) versus working with the mother toward the interests of the child, (such as a "good" mother tries to do what is good for her child).

All of these do's and don'ts, found through experience, may sound like platitudes or truisms upon first inspection. However, in practice they have been found to be the most difficult for the beginning dyadic psychotherapists to deal with when working with a dyad. For example, it is easy to promote unwittingly the idea that a mother should be the caretaker of her child. It is in fact a social value that is widely ascribed to. Yet when working with a severely disturbed mother who is emotionally incapable, even marginally, of taking care of herself, it is a disservice to the mother, and to her child, for the therapist to be unaware of his/her injection of this value onto the therapeutic intervention, and it makes it much more difficult for the mother to consider her options in reality.

SOME QUESTIONS AND ANSWERS

What is the importance of assessment of the infant?

The primary importance of assessing the infant is to determine whether there are any problems with the infant. Developmental delays, sensory, or motoric problems are important to be aware of. For one thing, the mother hopes and expects the baby to be essentially perfect. Any deviations from that will be a disappointment to her. The therapist needs to be aware of such deviations in order to deal more effectively with the mother's feelings around that. Also, the presence of any developmental delays or other problems may indicate the need for specific interventions in order to moderate them. These interventions are best begun as early as possible. If there is a suspicion concerning any problems intrinsic to the infant at birth, it is well to be aware of them in order to deal with them, in terms of both the baby and the reaction of the mother. Her emotions in dealing with her reaction and the consequent development of her interaction patterns with her baby must also be dealt with. In most cases, unless there has been illicit drug use, or medication, during pregnancy, the babies of the disturbed mother do not evidence developmental lags or problems at birth.

What is the importance of doing an assessment of the mother prior to beginning therapy?

The more knowledge the therapist has about the mother, the more effectively the therapist can understand her and apply the general orientation of the therapy to this mother and plan a therapeutic program for her. For most categories of psychopathology, this will mean the specific psychodynamic approach taken in the intervention. However, for particular cases, which are perhaps more serious or are in particular diagnostic categories, planning in terms of the mother's possible relapse is indicated.

Why is it important to assess the interaction between mother and baby?

The first observations of a mother interacting with her baby tend to predict the future. Therefore, the therapist must take microscopic views of the behavior pattern in the interactions seriously. The therapist needs to assess and weigh them in order to formulate a diagnostic impression of the pattern and to plan for therapeutic interventions. To a great extent, the expectations the mother has of the child will set the stage, either positively or negatively, for her manner of interacting with that child.

How are fathers included in the intervention?

Frequently the mother is the one who has made the therapy contact. In that case, if the father is willing to come to therapy and the mother agrees to his participation, then he is invited to come. Once the father is brought to the session, an assessment is made of his desire, willingness, and need to participate, and a plan is formulated for him as well. There are many possibilities. For example, the mother may not want her mate to participate in the therapy. She may be possessive about the therapy situation and want to keep it for herself and her baby. More typically, the mother will want the father to participate in the therapy and will invite him to come, if he is part of the household. If the father has distanced himself and is no longer a part of the household, in a supportive or loving relationship with the mother and/or child, then typically the woman will not desire him there. The participation of the father varies greatly. It varies from coming only once to being the "mothering person" or main nurturer of the infant and main participant in the dyadic psychotherapy. He may want to be very much involved with the baby or may be very much preoccupied with other things in his life at this time. The decision as to how to involve the father will need to be made taking these factors into account. There are several variations of how the father might be involved. He might require his own individual psychotherapy, which would require individual sessions for him. He might require dyadic sessions with the baby, perhaps alternating with the mother's sessions, or do so occasionally. It might be best for the family to have triadic sessions, that is, both parents and the baby in the same session.

What is the importance of involving significant others in the therapeutic interventions?

Significant others may have greater or lesser importance to the mother. For instance, if it is a single mother whose main emotional and perhaps other support comes from another family member (typically her mother), or another person such as a friend, it may be that this person needs to be involved in the same manner as a husband, as addressed in the previous question. Alternatively, it may be that the significant other is a secondary type of support person, who nevertheless has great importance to the mother, either directly in a day-to-day situation or at a greater distance in helping her to plan, being a kind of base or safety net for the mother. In that case, that person may be involved and made aware of the possibilities of greater need for her support at those times when the mother is less able to function well and to perform her motherly duties in a full fashion.

Under what circumstances are appropriate community agencies contacted in the treatment of the mother?

The greater the emotional disturbance of the mother, the greater is the likelihood that there will be additional problems which put the mother and her family at risk. These problems could include educational, vocational, financial, social, medical, substance abuse problems, and possibly others. The dyadic psychotherapy deals specifically in psychotherapeutically aiding in the development of a positive attachment or relationship between the mother and her baby. It cannot magically transform the total life of the mother. Consequently, when there are other problems, which put the mother and her family at risk or disadvantage, it is appropriate to enlist whatever support and help can be found for her or that she can be encouraged to find for herself in the community. The first step in this is to determine the problem areas, which can be done jointly between the therapist and the mother. For example, if there is substance abuse, it is absolutely imperative for the mother to be simultaneously in drug abuse treatment and to abstain from taking drugs, otherwise not only is she unable to function vis-à-vis the baby, but also she cannot benefit from the psychotherapeutic interventions, which are focused on her relationship with her baby. Similarly, if we have an extreme situation where there is chronically no food in the house, it is not possible to do remedial work in such circumstances. Under this kind of duress, the mother will not be able to focus her attention. The primary needs will have to be met. The same holds for vocational lacks. In that situation, though the urgency will not be as great, the mother's total development to be able to function effectively as a person is important. For instance, as a single mother, she will need to develop some skills that will allow her to work independently.

Why does the mother's immaturity create problems?

The "normal" mature woman has developed to a point beyond being self-centered and egocentric. She has gone beyond having the main focus of her psyche being self-development, reaching emotional maturity, and exerting efforts toward figuring out how to interact with other people. She has some sense of security and wholeness within herself, being able to be relatively unselfconscious in her interactions with other people, is able to be task-oriented, has a philosophy of life that guides her in the minutia of everyday living, has developed her sense of morality and ethics, has accumulated a fair amount of information about the world, has an interest in what goes on around her, and has a sense of participation in the society in which she lives. The person who has not come to this point is still striving to get there, and has this achievement as her goal. She will tend to be egocentric, concerned with herself, be preoccupied with all of the unresolved issues, conflicts, and the development of a style of life, which are appropriate to her level of maturity, which most typically is related to the age of that person. The amount of interest and energy devoted to others is more limited. When that other is her own baby, who is dependent upon her, she will fail to give that baby the full attention and emotional warmth that the baby requires for optimal development.

What are the problems created by older motherhood?

Older does not mean more mature but rather approaching aging. In that sense, the older mother has as her task for that level of development things other than motherhood. She has to come to terms with aging, decreased speed of reactivity, and decreased speed of functioning in many areas of her life. She has to deal with losses of previous children leaving home and to cope with functions that she has performed in the past that are now either diminishing or being relinquished. To the extent that the woman is dealing with those losses, it is less appropriate to mother a child. She cannot focus her energies as well on previous developmental tasks related to child rearing, which she has already outlived and which are no longer appropriate to her.

What is the importance, to the very disturbed mother, of experiencing the therapist as competent to deal with her extremely strong fears and impulses?

The person who has extremely strong fears and impulses is disturbed by them. They tend to be hovering just near awareness, and affect all of her functioning. She will be afraid of not having control in relation to these. If they are strong, she will feel as though the very impulses can be harmful to others, including the therapist. If the therapist is not aware of this, and is intimidated and afraid of the patient's impulses in the therapy session, this will keep the patient from being able to relate in a way that is therapeutic. This will tend to increase the anxiety around these impulses and fears. On the other hand, the disturbed mother who feels that the therapist is competent enough to deal with her strong impulses will then be able to relax and have confidence in herself not to express these, and thereby be able to focus on doing the necessary therapeutic work.

What is meant here by a supportive approach in the therapeutic relationship?

The therapeutic approach equals the feeling on the part of the patient that the therapist is trying to understand her and is able to do so at least part of the time. This understanding is communicated to the patient by the therapist's reflection of feelings that are, at least part of the time, on target, by an understanding communicated by the therapist of what underlies the symptoms, and by the therapist's interpretation of the psychodynamics of the patient, which are on target, at least some of the time. In other words, the mother feels emotionally supported by the therapist because she feels that the therapist tries to, and in fact does, understand her, at least to some extent. The mother with a young child offers a special opportunity to the therapist to use supportive interventions in the sense that the interventions can be based on the observed emotional and behavioral interactions between mother and child. Furthermore, the mother is particularly appreciative of these interventions because she experiences that they are helpful to her in understanding and/or positively interacting with her baby.

What would be an example of interpretation of mother-infant interactions?

The concept is to observe the behavioral interaction of mother and infant and at what points the therapist feels the mother's behavior is an expression of her psychodynamics rather than her attempts to meet the needs of the baby. The therapist makes an effort to understand what those psychodynamics are and verbalizes an interpretation of this. For instance, a mother with a two-month-old baby tries to put the baby's hands on the bottle while she is feeding him, in an effort to have him hold the bottle for himself, during the therapy session. The therapist might say: "You would like Johnny to hold his own bottle; you really would like him to be bigger already; you don't like him being helpless." If the mother registers this interpretation with some relief on her part, then it is probable that the therapist has, at least in part, made a valid interpretation. For instance, the therapist may have felt that this mother has an extreme ambivalence about having others depend on her, feeling herself to be incompetent, or possibly resentful of burdens put on her. Possibly, without her being aware of it, she wants the child not to be dependent on her, to be grown up and take care of itself. Once this is brought to the awareness of the mother, the likelihood is that she will realize that this is unrealistic and change her behavior to treat the baby as a baby, that is, at the appropriate age level, and hold the bottle for him.

What would be an example of an interpretation of the mother's transference interactions with her baby?

A mother who, let us say, is an extremely fearful person, identifies with her baby, and will project that her baby is also fearful, in her emotional transference interaction with her baby. In a therapy situation, for example, a mother may be fearful of noises and project that fear onto the baby. She may say, for instance, that the baby is afraid of any noise. This would tend to make her overprotective of the baby in relation to its exposure to noise. In the therapy situation, if the therapist is able to pick up on these projections and identify transference interactions, an interpretation can be made to the mother. For instance: "One of your problems is your fear of noises. When the baby startles at a noise, you feel as though he is also afraid of noises, just as you are. In fact, the reaction he just had to a noise was a startle response, which is a reflex reaction on the part of the baby. It does not mean that he is a fearful baby." The attempt here is twofold: to intercede in the mother's tendency to project the specific fear of noises onto the baby; and to help the mother to learn to differentiate herself from the baby, that they are not one and the same.

What is the purpose of the therapist's translating the infant's needs to the mother?

A mother who is apparently oblivious to the needs of her child will not be responsive to these needs. If this is the case, the probability is that she will continue to be oblivious, and that this will create a vicious cycle in the interaction between mother and child. For instance, if the baby looks uncomfortable in the mother's arms, the therapist might say something to the effect: "Mommy, I feel like I'm falling off your lap," thereby communicating to the mother, with the attempt to be non-threatening, the needs of the child. The mother is thereby made aware of the baby's needs and will tend then to meet them. This type of intervention will probably be required repeatedly, until the mother learns to focus more on the child. In the interim, she will not have lost sight of those needs and of meeting them.

What would be an example of modeling?

When a positive interactive behavior is lacking on the part of the mother, the therapist may resort to modeling as a technique. For instance, if there is very little attempt by the mother to talk to, or make sounds to, the baby, and the development of verbal interaction is missing or less than optimal, the therapist may make some sounds to the baby directly and engage the baby. The mother watching this tends to be intrigued and charmed, as well as somewhat envious in that the therapist has been able to elicit a fun interaction with the baby. The mother is then encouraged to do this herself. She will tend to follow through and gain the fun of the interaction herself with the baby. With some mothers this will take a good deal of repetition, but there is a tendency to learn the interaction because it is rewarding to experience the fun in doing so. It is also a good idea for the therapist to reflect the feeling that the mother is having fun in this interaction.

What would be an example of behavioral directives?

Behavioral directives are used as sparingly as possible. Since mothers typically resent being told what to do, behavioral directives are kept at a minimum. They are typically used only after other techniques have been tried and have not ameliorated the lack of or negative interaction with the baby. For instance, if there is a lack of verbal interaction with the child, and other techniques have been tried, including modeling, to no avail, then the therapist might say to the mother: "Now talk to the baby," giving this specific directive to her. Or, if the mother does not make eye contact with the baby, the therapist might say: "Look at your baby, look in her eyes. You see she's looking back at you," and thereby try to start a cycle of interaction through eye contact. Behavioral directives are also given in emergencies. If the mother's behavior, or her lack of action, is putting the baby at risk, behavioral directives are appropriate. For instance, if the baby is about to fall off the dressing table, and the mother is nearby but not watching, the therapist at a distance might say: "Hold the baby," or "Put your hand on the baby," in order to avoid a catastrophe. This is particularly important, not only because the catastrophe will thus be avoided, but also because the mother understands through this that the therapist cares enough to have given this directive and did not display a lack of caring by allowing the mother to be negligent enough to allow the baby to fall.

6

Dyadic Psychotherapy Interventions: Types and Examples

Some typical types of interventions used by the therapist in dyadic psychotherapy are illustrated in this chapter through examples of cases. In particular, seven major types of therapeutic interventions are noted. They cover interactions such as putting the infant's reaction into words for the mother, the reflection of feelings, the making of interpretations, and the modeling of infant behaviors for the parent. Intervention in the interest of the child is, and continues to be, the key factor in the rationale of the treatment process.

Establishing and maintaining a psychodynamic therapeutic alliance, in general, depends on the extent to which the client feels that she is empathically understood by the therapist and that there is hope for relief of the psychic pain suffered. In dyadic psychotherapy, the psychodynamics of the therapeutic alliance are complicated by the infant and by the mother's feelings about it. The mother generally wants good things for her baby. The emotionally disturbed mother, however, tends to expect the infant to meet her own emotional needs, which have been so painfully unfulfilled. The infant is unable to supply what is needed by the mother. The mother has, therefore, already been disappointed in the infant in that she, the mother, has not received nurturance from the infant. Since typically the emotionally disturbed mother is also either emotionally, or actually, separated from other adults (husband, mother, other family members), she has usually lacked the satisfaction of other people's admiration for her baby, and the consequent reflection of her own achievement in having brought this wonderful new life into the world. This mother is therefore unable to see herself reflected in her baby or to experience joy in relation to it. The therapist needs to counteract this lack in order to form a therapeutic alliance and help the mother with her attachment to the infant.

TYPICAL INTERVENTIONS

Therapist's Expression of Admiration, Sympathy, and Understanding

The therapist needs to express admiration and enthusiasm for the infant. This enables the mother to look at her infant through the eyes of the therapist. As a result she may then be able to admire the baby for the first time and perhaps experience some joy in doing so.

For example, when Linda brought her baby for the first time, she sat on the couch with her baby across her lap in the "log effect," waiting for her therapist. Linda expressed no emotion, nor did she look down at her baby. When the therapist entered, Linda timidly waited for the therapist to interact with her. The therapist came in, looked at the baby with a broad smile, and said, "What a wonderful baby you have, Mommy!" "Look at him, Mommy! He's so cute!" At this, Linda looked down at her baby and started to participate in admiring him. It seemed that, for the first time, she saw him as something special and took satisfaction in the reflected glory. The therapist then asked how the delivery had gone, and expressed sympathy and understanding for the difficulties involved.

As the therapy progresses, other therapeutic interventions will be brought into play.

Rewarding Positive Mothering Behaviors and Affects

When the mother displays behavior directly or indirectly beneficial to the child, the therapist provides the mother with rewards. The reward is most frequently verbalization, but it may also be a facial expression, non-verbal sound, or postural reaction. Disturbed mothers typically use positive mothering behaviors sparsely. Consequently the therapist needs to have patience in waiting for these to emerge.

For example, after several sessions, Mary had not yet achieved eye contact with her baby. She avoided looking in her baby's eyes. She was busy inspecting his ears, brushing his hair, and cleaning his nose. All of these behaviors were experienced by the baby as intrusive; he looked uncomfortable and made avoidant movements. The therapist, in sympathy with the baby, was also feeling uncomfortable with Mary's intrusiveness but said nothing. She feared that a negative remark would work against the feebly developing therapeutic alliance. Mary sat quietly, and then fleetingly looked into the baby's eyes. He returned her gaze. Mary's facial expression remained impassive. The therapist said, "Oh! He's looking back at you." Mary returned to her eye contact with him. She smiled.

Putting the Infant's Reaction into Words for the Mother

Continuing with the above session, the therapist said: "The baby likes it when you look in his eyes."

Reflection of Feelings

And "You like it when he looks at you. It's so nice that you're enjoying him." Mary continued the eye contact. She gradually became aware of her own pleasure, and took satisfaction in this awareness.

In subsequent sessions Mary was able to look into the baby's eyes more readily. However, she continued her intrusive behavior toward the baby. The therapist now felt that the therapeutic alliance was sufficiently well developed to allow for a limited focus on negative behaviors. When Mary picked at the baby's ear and he squirmed, the therapist verbalized for the baby: "Mommy, I don't like that" ("Putting the Infant's Reaction into Words for the Mother," as in the intervention above). Mary stopped the picking. She repeated intrusive behaviors in many later sessions. However, with continued interventions, she was able to develop empathy for the child. She significantly diminished her intrusiveness.

Interpretations

Though the object of the therapy is not the mother as an individual, there is a strong therapeutic alliance. Furthermore, the therapist, from the beginning, has made a strong effort to know the mother—her life-style, defenses, and psychodynamics—well. Thus, there may be opportunities for incisive interpretations of the mother's dynamics during the therapy process.

For example, Jane has been in dyadic psychotherapy for six months. During this time she has, on occasion, expressed her anxiety about her own confused, bizarre thinking. For instance, Jane's mother gave her strange dictates as to how she should treat her baby. She thought these dictates were wrong and strange, and did not want to carry them out. She was, however, confused by them because she lacked confidence in her own perceptions and opinions. She was therefore in conflict. She generally felt compelled to carry out the dictates of her mother and, on the other hand, felt that it was wrong or illogical to do so. She interpreted her confusion as "crazy."

In one session she said she had had a dream about her cousin. She then related how her cousin had died when she was a little girl. Jane had been fond of this cousin, did not understand death, and felt the loss severely. At the funeral she looked into the coffin. She said: "My cousin winked at me." This was told to the therapist in a confused way, within the context of her feeling "crazy." The therapist, using the therapeutic alliance, with great empathy, and well aware of the psychodynamics involved, said: "You loved your cousin. You did not want him to die. You wished him alive. And so, you felt as though he winked at you." Jane's face cleared. She looked as though an enormous weight had been lifted from her. The feeling of "craziness" she had been plagued with, remarkably, did not recur.

Modeling

Though the therapist waits for positive mothering behaviors in order to reward them, in some cases these do not appear spontaneously.

Ida, after several months of dyadic psychotherapy, had been able to establish eye contact and develop empathy for her newborn baby. However, she continued to be non-verbal toward him. She did not coo to him, did not indulge in baby talk, nor did she talk to him. The therapist decided to use modeling as a technique of intervention. The therapist turned to the baby and directly engaged him in making sounds, smiling and looking in his eyes. He reciprocated, and an interchange ensued. The therapist and the baby had fun in this. Ida watched. With some encouragement, Ida too then participated in a dialogue with her baby. The therapist made her aware of her own pleasure in this ("Reflection of Feelings"). After this technique had been used over a series of sessions, Ida became somewhat more spontaneous in her verbal interplay with her baby, which made it possible for the therapist increasingly to use reward as an intervention for the verbal behaviors ("Rewarding Positive Mothering Behavior and Affects").

Behavioral Directives

Behavioral directives are generally not used in dyadic psychotherapy. They are reserved only for crises and for particularly cogent situations.

Example of a crisis: If a child is in danger of being hurt (e.g., falling), fast action is required. It is inappropriate to allow the child to get hurt. Aside from the physical harm to the child, the therapist's neutrality or laissez-faire attitude would also signal the mother that the therapist does not care. The mother might also gain additional odd ideas from such laissez-faire behavior, for example, that she herself is blameless if the child is hurt and/or that the child should be able to take care of itself.

Example of a cogent situation: Linda held her one-month-old infant in her arms. She looked down at him pensively for some time. She then said to the therapist, "I hate to think of when he gets older and I have to hit him." In this statement she was saying that she felt it was necessary for a mother to discipline her child through hitting and that even the thought made her feel bad. The therapist stated the behavioral directive: "Don't worry. You won't hit him." The therapist then explained: "Hitting hurts the child. It is not good for him. Also, you're already feeling bad about the idea of hitting him. It would only make you feel guilty." Linda looked relieved. In subsequent months she did not hit him. The topic did not reappear in the sessions for a year.

CONCLUSION

These seven types of therapeutic interventions are highly effective. Used selectively, sensitively, and empathically, as appropriate, the dyadic relationship is very much helped in its positive development. The mother increasingly interacts in a nurturing and contingent way, avoids irrational attributions to the infant, and increases her empathy for the child. She is also able to gain satisfaction and joy in her interactions. The child is able to benefit from appropriate infant care and to develop well emotionally, without major setbacks or the emergence and development of massive psychopathology.

This is also the case when the mother is so emotionally debilitated that she is unable to be a primary caretaker for her child. Through dyadic psychotherapy, and her increased empathy and clearer vision of her reality situation, she will be able to give higher priority to the interests of the child. She will therefore be more ready to allow the child to be cared for by others, who in this case are more capable of taking care of the child in a nurturing way.

SOME QUESTIONS AND ANSWERS

Is the therapist's expression of admiration, sympathy, and understanding unusual in a therapy situation?

It would be considered relatively unusual for the therapist to express these pointedly as part of the therapeutic intervention, within most individual therapies. In the context of dyadic psychotherapy, if the mother presents herself as displaying behavior that indicates a lack of interaction with her baby and an apathetic or distanced approach to the child, it is of prime importance for the therapist to try to affect the mother's emotional and behavioral interaction with her baby from the very beginning. Mothers' deep emotional feelings concerning their infants are assumed by the therapist. If the therapist were to fail to try to impact this lack of interaction between the two, the mother would interpret that as a rejection of herself as well as of her baby. She would then tend to see the therapist as similar to the other rejecting figures in her life. She has already experienced them as rejecting of her pregnancy and of the baby itself. Expression of admiration for a baby is a natural reaction of adults who are not constrained by emotional problems. It is important for the therapist to allow him/herself to express this reaction.

Why might therapists find it problematic to express admiration for the baby?

The beginning dyadic psychotherapist tends not to find it natural for a therapist to express admiration to a patient. They have typically learned to assume a more passive stance in the interactions with their clients. They have learned to curb the direct expressions of their own emotional reactions to their clients. They therefore find this intervention novel, and need to accustom themselves to it.

What is another difficulty for the beginning dyadic psychotherapist?

It is very difficult for a nurturing person to witness less than nurturing behavior toward a baby. The impulse is to intervene directly. When a baby cries, and the mother does not soothe it, the impulse is to soothe the baby directly. Standing by and being witness to the lack of nurturing and gentle stimulation are typically extremely difficult for all therapists.

What is the importance of the therapist not playing a direct nurturing role with the baby?

If the therapist starts to nurture the baby him/herself, the mother will see this as a criticism. She will feel reinforced in the idea that she is incapable of caring for that baby. She will therefore either withdraw further from the care of the baby or become angry at the therapist. In either case, the therapeutic process has taken some steps backwards as a result.

In the case of the mother who tends not to make eye contact, how is it that the therapist can sit and wait for this to happen?

Even though the mother tends not to make eye contact, in fact avoids it, in most instances sooner or later there will be a fleeting glance at the baby within the session. If the baby is alert at that moment, it will react to the mother's eye contact. It is possible to wait for this to happen, allowing the natural eye contact to take place, though momentarily, and to capitalize on this interaction.

Why does the therapist put the infant's reactions into words for the mother?

To the degree that the mother has a disturbance, she tends to be preoccupied with herself. She therefore tends to be thinking about herself rather than how other people might feel. This includes the baby. She tends not to think of the baby's feelings. Therefore, if the therapist puts the baby's reactions into words, the mother's attention is drawn in that direction. She will then be able to pay attention to the baby's feelings. This will likely be very fleeting. However, with repeated interventions of this sort, the mother will begin to be able to put herself in the place of the baby, attempting to read or guess at the feelings the baby may be having. In other words, she will start to develop empathy.

Why does the therapist seek to have the mother enjoy her baby?

Enjoying one's baby is the natural course of events in the normal mother-child relationship. It is the natural reward that the mother receives. It consequently functions as a motivator to continue to act in such a way as to continue to receive the pleasurable responses of the child. This equals interacting with the child in a considered, empathic manner and in the interests of the child.

What makes the mother's negative behaviors toward the child particularly difficult for the therapist to deal with?

Interventions that directly impact the mother's negative behaviors toward the baby are most likely experienced as punitive and rejecting. This goes counter and is destructive to the therapeutic alliance, unless that alliance is well established and interventions concerning negative behaviors are carefully couched and used sparingly.

When should modeling be used as an intervention?

Two reasons for cautiousness in using modeling are: (1) it is behavior initiated by the therapist rather than by the mother; and (2) it can be seen by the client as criticism. On the other hand, modeling is often effective in initiating behavior that does not seem to be spontaneously forthcoming in the mother's interactions with the child. If the therapist feels that it is important at this time of development of the infant for the mother to engage in certain interactions with the baby, then she may bring in the intervention of modeling. The exact timing of the use of modeling is a judgment call on the part of the therapist.

Why is it that behavioral directives are generally not used in dyadic psychotherapy?

Directives to the mother tend to be experienced as criticism of her. Most disturbed women feel that they have not been allowed to develop their own directions and to take charge of their own lives. They therefore tend to resent people telling them what to do. Very frequently they will become oppositional and will frustrate the therapist. Although there are exceptions, behavioral directives are therefore generally counterindicated.

7

Case Studies of the Most Severely
Disturbed Dyads: Applying
Dyadic Psychotherapy Theory
and Findings to the
Understanding and Treatment
of Dyads

This chapter explores what happens when the understandings, theory, concepts, and findings noted in chapters 3 and 4 are applied to infants and parents. Illustrative worst case scenarios of psychotic mothers are presented here. These refer to and represent each of the four types of psychotic mothers discussed earlier in chapter 3.

It is clear from the illustrations that the behavior emanating from the psychodynamic process of schizophrenia is quite disparate, particularly depending upon whether it is paranoid schizophrenia or not. This latter category is here labeled non-paranoid schizophrenia, to designate those forms of schizophrenia other than the paranoid type. This difference between types is found to be highlighted, especially in the mothering behavior (see chapter 4).

Each case is presented concisely, giving a description of the mother, her distinctive ideation, and her mothering reactions, and of the resultant impact and formation of developmental characteristics in the child.

TYPE 1. PREDOMINANTLY NON-PARANOID TYPE OF SCHIZOPHRENIA IN THE MOTHER

Eileen was in her mid-twenties. She had never made an adequate adjustment to life (Schizotypal Personality Disorder, previously called Simple Schizophrenia). She had done very poorly academically as well, and was unprepared for the work world.

Her high level of fear prevented her from interacting with others. Though she was in need of a sense of connectedness with others, her emotional isolation was well practiced and generalized. She was unable to make an effort to have her needs met. This resulted in an overlay of depression. She appeared sluggish, was unkempt, spoke hardly at all, and then in a slurred, inarticulate manner. She typically displayed no affect nor reciprocity. She took no initiative, and generally interacted minimally with others, including her children.

Eileen did not look in her baby Serena's eyes. She did not hold and cradle her baby. She did not coo or talk to Serena. In fact, her interactions with her infant were typified by their absence.

Her anxiety mainfested itself in nervous movements. This included frequently removing the baby bottle from Serena, making feeding difficult. During the sessions, Eileen would put Serena across her lap in the "log effect." Since Eileen was highly guarded, she did not reveal her bizarre thinking (which was evidenced on psychological testing). Unrealistic expectations can be summarized in her having the idea that she needed to do essentially nothing for the baby.

The neglect this infant truly experienced was highlighted through a structured interview concerning her daily life, the "Typical Day Interview" (see Appendix E). It evidenced that at home Serena was typically in bed or on the floor, that is, not in contact with Eileen. Eileen already wanted Serena, at two months of age, to hold her own bottle.

Eileen put Serena in a walker at seven months, although the child was clearly not ready for this, in order to ease her burden of taking care of her. On a typical day, Eileen claimed not to say one word to Serena, not to play with her, not to cuddle her, and not to pick her up. Her interactions with the child were minimal.

Eileen and her two children lived in her mother's home. Though her mother and her mother's husband were present each evening, there was little interchange with Eileen, and essentially none with Serena.

Serena was normal at birth. At two months of age she was in the average range on testing (Bayley Scales of Infant Development). However, her level of functioning declined with age. By seven months her scores had dipped significantly. Eileen and Serena had stopped coming to sessions. Serena's scores declined further by one year, as evidenced at a visit. By two years the scores were extremely low (scoring in the lowest first percentile in both mental and motor scales). Serena did not grow well physically; by two years she was small for her age. She also lacked clear eye contact, and was delayed in speech and in both gross and fine motor development.

Eileen had liked coming to the sessions. These met some of her needs for attention. She produced little spontaneous behavior which would lend itself to therapeutic intervention. Consequently suggestions to the mother were utilized to a greater extent than usual. (Typically, suggestions are a last resort in the choice of interventions.) She would try to comply momentarily to a given intervention, and did seem to gain a slight degree of pleasure from these orchestrated interactions with her baby.

Eileen, however, remained mainly apathetic and anhedonic. She discontinued coming to sessions after a short time. Alternative group sessions were offered her, which she also chose not to attend.

TYPE 2. PARANOID SCHIZOPHRENIA IN THE MOTHER

The behavior of the mother in interacting with her infant will depend upon the specific mixture of levels of fear, anxiety, depression, and defenses, as well as the nature of the ideational content.

Case 1

Joan, twenty-five years old, had a high level of denied fear of the world and of her own aggressive impulses. However, her anxiety level was so high that she tended to freeze and therefore to interact minimally with her infant. When she did interact, it was in a stereotyped, rigid manner. Because of the freezing, she tended not to stimulate the infant; intrusive stimulation was also lacking. In fact, she sat with the baby across her lap in the "log effect." The baby's head hung down off her lap, on one side, while the feet did the same on the other. At rest, Joan did not hold the baby in her arms, nor talk to or look at her. She was also depressed, which tended to reduce her interactions as well.

Joan had had several stays in mental hospitals. She was a late, and only, child of an elderly couple. Her father was bedridden, chronically ill, and in his eighties. Her mother, also in her eighties, was his caretaker; she was feeble and had difficulty walking.

Emphasis had been placed, by these elderly parents, on Joan's education. She had attended college briefly. She spoke well and performed capably in her "office" behavior. However, Joan was not capable of caring for her baby. She had lost custody of the child due to neglect. Joan was, at this time, living with her parents, who had custody of the child. Joan's mother was overburdened with a business enterprise she had of day care for infants and toddlers. Consequently Joan did a good deal of helping to take care of her own baby, as well as of the other children in her mother's care.

Unfortunately, Joan's delusional system started to include her baby. Her "voices" told her to take the infant to the zoo and feed her to the lions. Joan was able to resist the "voices" only partially. It was the middle of winter, but she did take the child to the zoo. However, she did not follow through on the command to feed her to the lions. During the next night, though, the baby woke up hungry. Joan took her and carried her to the kitchen. On the way she "walked into a door jamb." The result was a subdural hematoma for the baby. The child's injury affected her development, which was consequently delayed. The mother then came to therapy. The therapist worked to help sustain Joan through the rehabilitative therapy offered the infant elsewhere.

In this case, a set of unfortunate circumstances produced injury to the child. Joan's severe anxiety and generalized diminished activity level reduced her positive symptoms; consequently the intrusive behavior, which is typical of the paranoid schizophrenic mother, was also not noted. Her involving paranoid ideation, however, put the child at high risk.

Case 2

Peggy, thirty-two years old, had two previous children who had been placed, from birth on, with out-of-town relatives. Her youngest, a two-year-old, was in protective custody in a foster home. Peggy had been hospitalized. She was doing better and was living independently. She wanted to regain custody of her child. Two-year-old Tommy met his mother at a therapy session after almost two years of separation. He was a small, shy little boy. He was reticent to touch any toys in the play room. His interactions with his mother and the therapist were also limited. He shied away from both. Peggy was disturbed by this "rejecting" behavior. She wanted to interact with Tommy. She therefore started to put crayon to paper. She told him to draw a circle. After a while he accomplished this. Peggy was not satisfied with its quality. She criticized the circle and tried to have him draw again in order to perfect it. Shy Tommy reacted to the criticism with further withdrawal. Peggy became more frustrated and angry.

During the ensuing sessions, Peggy demonstrated her intrusiveness in her inspections of Tommy's ears, eyes, and scalp, all of which were annoying to Tommy. She also tried to direct his behavior in a rigid, stereotyped manner. For instance, sitting behind Tommy, she would lock Tommy between her legs, as he was playing on a low table, or she would place her hand over his as he was trying to draw or play on a xylophone, controlling his movements.

Since depression was low, it did not inhibit her behavior. Her paranoid ideation centered about her employer and her landlord, as well as her friends. It did not involve Tommy. Consequently the worst aspect of the interactions was the intrusive, rigid behavior. Peggy was able to benefit from the dyadic psychotherapy and to relinquish some of the overcontrolling and intrusive behaviors. She continued to want custody of Tommy and to work toward it. Tommy experienced her sustained interest and love for him, and he began to attach to her. His behavior improved. He became less shy and interacted well with Peggy. He now came over to her during the sessions in order to involve her in his play. The relationship was going so well that Tommy was allowed to go on home visits with Peggy, at first for the day and then for weekends.

Peggy, however, had difficulty in controlling his now less inhibited behavior. She tended to allow him to do anything, not wanting to alienate him by saying "no." Tommy needed age-appropriate controls. Before Peggy was able to master this, Tommy was given to her for a prolonged time as a "test" of primary caretaking capability by the foster care agency, contrary to the therapist's recommendation. Though she was delighted, Peggy was not ready for this. Within several weeks, she became very disturbed, felt incapable of handling him, and consequently became extremely angry and hostile. She refused further treatment. Soon Tommy was removed from her care and had to be returned to his foster home.

Tommy nevertheless had gained an attachment to his mother and the feeling that she (someone) cared deeply about him. He consequently had achieved an improved self-image and a greater freedom to develop.

Peggy had also developed an attachment to her son, as well as a positive manner of interacting with him, which brought mutual satisfaction to both. However, she suffered greatly from the attempt to move toward reunion too quickly.

These two cases illustrate common factors in paranoid schizophrenics' interactions with their infants. They also illustrate the vast differences that can be found depending upon the specific mix of factors affecting the behavior. In one case, there was an involving delusion of the infant. In the other case, the infant was not involved in the delusional system. In the first case, the mother's activity level was diminished due to high levels of anxiety and depression, which consequently also diminished intrusive behavior. In the second, this was not the case; intrusive behavior predominated. Therefore, in the first case the child was at high risk for injury, while in the second situation this was not the case, but rather there was a risk for development of rigid-conforming behavior (which was effectively ameliorated through the dyadic psychotherapy).

TYPE 3. BIPOLAR DISORDER IN THE MOTHER

Case 1

Carla, twenty-one years old, was in her third trimester of pregnancy. She was on her sixth admission to a mental hospital. She had recently quit her job because she felt her boss was unreasonable. Carla's mother lived in the area. She was, however, not a support to Carla. She would not allow Carla to live with her in her apartment. Carla said her mother drank and sought out Carla to ask for money. Carla's father had died in a mental hospital. Carla had a five-year-old son for whom she had not been caretaker. He lived in the South with relatives. The father of the present baby had asked her to marry him, but she was glad that she had not done so. She said that she was better off without him. She did continue to have a relationship with him, however. He intended to visit the baby, and she planned to use the father's last name for the baby.

Her diagnosis of bipolar affective disorder was displayed classically in her mood swings. During her hypomanic phase she had lots of ideas, wrote poetry, made plans for her life, and moved about quite a bit. During this period of her life she fluctuated between in- and out-patient status many times.

Carla had been living in shelters and had hoped to find housing during the latter part of her pregnancy. She never succeeded in this. The baby was born one month prematurely; consequently she had no place of her own when the baby arrived. Mother and baby therefore lived in hotels and rooming houses, where she had no kitchen facilities. It was not possible for her to sterilize the baby's bottles. Carla was also an expert at irritating people, and therefore managed to be evicted repeatedly. At these times she called the police so that her baby would be cared for. Protective services would then take the baby.

Carla did take care of the baby's needs in feeding and changing. What characterized Carla, however, was that she was always busy meeting her own needs. During therapy sessions she was preoccupied in trying to gain the approval of the therapist, and so she spent most of her attention and energies in talking and interacting with her. Consequently, eye contact with her infant was highly limited. Vestibular stimulation occurred only tangentially to the mother's own movements. Tactual stimulation occurred tangentially. There was no evidence of soothing or molding. Auditory stimulation occurred tangentially (she did not talk or make noises directly to baby).

Typically, Carla paid little attention to her baby as she struggled to maintain her position on her mother's lap. She did place her hand on the baby when she bent over to pick up something from the floor, in order to keep her from falling. When the therapist left the room, Carla sat still, staring ahead of her. She did not interact with the baby. On the therapist's return she became extremely occupied with removing items from the baby bag, which had become wet from spills of a baby bottle. Carla was busy wiping the "sterile" bottle liners and other paraphernalia. When she decided to change the baby, she did it still busily talking to the therapist, without particular regard to the baby while changing her. She left her unguarded on the changing table when she went to fetch something. When Carla decided to give the baby her bottle, she stated that there was water in it, saying the baby was not hungry. It turned out that though she had some baby formula in her bag, she did not have a can opener and so could not use it. The therapist located and sterilized a can opener for her. Carla dropped it on the floor before opening the can.

The baby was not able to catch her mother's eye and in fact tended to turn away from her (gaze aversion). The baby's cries did not elicit a response on the part of the mother; at one month, the baby had already learned not to cry. There was a minimum of vocalization of any kind. The baby's experience was that her actions did not produce a reaction in her mother. She was not capable of effectively producing a reaction in her mother to having her needs met. She had learned to be passive and that she could not help herself. The baby did appear alert. It can be interpreted that she was passive, though vigilantly awaiting gratification.

Case 2

Geraldine was a twenty-five-year-old mother of three young children. The older two were permanently placed with out-of-town relatives. The youngest, two-year-old Betsy, was in foster care. She had been removed because of neglect.

Geraldine had been hospitalized several times in the last few years. Her behavior with Betsy had earlier been noted as interpersonally distant. She had not adequately dressed nor fed her at age one month.

At two years Betsy was a delicate, compliant child, small for her age. She was friendly, smiled, and interacted nicely with others. Geraldine was happy to see Betsy in the therapy session, after almost two years of separation. She was extremely active with the child, suggesting one activity after another. After a half hour Geraldine was at a loss as to what to do next. The child's moment-to-moment needs escaped Geraldine. She was busy intrusively imposing her ideas of activities for the two of them.

At first she tried hard to interact with Betsy and also with the therapist. Across several sessions, however, she became more blatantly occupied with meeting her own needs. She brought food for herself and spent her hour eating it, or brought rock music for herself to listen to.

After a series of sessions, Geraldine did have the insight to realize that she was emotionally incapable of taking care of Betsy. This insight was made clear when she herself suggested giving Betsy up for adoption.

TYPE 4. MAJOR DEPRESSION IN THE MOTHER

Case 1

Rose, thirty-four years old, had lost custody of her two children due to neglect. Her older child, a four-year-old boy, was being cared for by relatives, and her one-and-a-half-year-old daughter had been placed in an orphanage. Rose had become extremely depressed after a death in the family, had then lost her job, and had been hospitalized. After a year she was feeling somewhat improved. She started in dyadic psychotherapy with her toddler, Kim. Her depression kept her from reaching out actively to the toddler. Her tendency was to sit passively watching Kim and feeling rejected by her. Rose was hoping that Kim would approach her. Kim, however, had already developed serious problems and was herself depressed. Due to the prolonged separation between mother and child, Kim did not remember Rose. Kim was not attached to her mother, nor was Rose attached to Kim. Through the therapy an attachment soon developed.

Both were then able to reach out to each other. Rose was pleased when Kim started to come to her, and Kim was pleased by her mother's attention. Their attachment for each other developed well. Rose did not have the same attachment problems with the older child, Kerry, since that had been previously established and was remembered. Kerry, however, was small for his age and quiet. Rose worried about him. She herself was improving clinically and was able to live at home. She regained custody of her children. Rose tried hard to be a good mother. Her depression interfered, so that she had to struggle to keep up her energy. Her guilt feelings also interfered with her assertiveness. She consequently was not able to use her resources as well as she might have been able to do otherwise. However, she did complete a vocational training course and obtained a position. Rose was now taking care of her children.

With her own improvement, Rose had been able to regain custody of her children. Her increased positive attachment to them, and more child-oriented, less self-centered, interaction with the children, allowed them to develop freer interaction patterns and to make good adjustments both interpersonally and academically. Rose had been able to effect giving the children the attention and support they needed in order to enable them to develop adequately.

Case 2

Brenda was a twenty-seven-year-old mother of two children. She had been in a mental hospital for several months. Her children had previously been removed from her custody because of neglect. After that, she and their father had been homeless for several months. Her psychotic breakdown had culminated when she had been told that all members of her family would die if she did not bring them all to religious services, which she was unable to do. The central role of guilt feelings in major depression is illustrated by this.

Both children, one-and-a-half-year-old Linda and two-and-a-half-year-old Johnny, had been placed with a foster family for a year. They had been able to make a satisfactory adjustment there. A reunion session of Brenda and her two children took place within the therapy. Linda had no memory of her mother. She approached her as a stranger. Johnny reacted timidly, a bit taken aback at first. Afterwards, he was very careful and vigilant in relation to his mother. Brenda was happy to see her children. She was careful in her approach to them; she tried to play with them in a gentle non-intrusive manner. When they became involved with a toy, Brenda withdrew into silently reading a children's book to herself or playing with toys herself. It seemed she was defending herself against feelings of rejection by the children.

The children remained in the foster home. In the therapy, as their relationship grew over time, Brenda tried harder to initiate interactions with the children. She tried doing this in a "playful" manner. Unfortunately her only mode was through teasing them and then laughing. Through therapeutic interventions, she gradually acquired other ways of interacting with them and was, to a large extent, able to abandon the teasing.

Linda's attachment to her mother developed smoothly over a period of months, in the hour-per-week sessions. Johnny had more difficulty in reestablishing an attachment. A good deal of anger expressed itself in his interactions with Brenda. This appeared to be a residual from earlier experiences. Dyadic sessions were instituted; Brenda was now seen twice

a week, once with each child. This was done in order to help Johnny and
Brenda to develop positive attachment and to allow Johnny to work
through the angry feelings. They all benefited greatly from this. Brenda
was later able to regain employment and an apartment, and then finally
the custody of her children. She later informed the therapist that she now
realized that the more love she gave the children, the easier they were to
care for.

8

The Length of Treatment in Dyadic Psychotherapy

This chapter discusses issues concerning the length of treatment, using dyadic psychotherapy, which may last from a few sessions for "average" mothers up to two or more years of intensive treatment for emotionally disturbed parents. Problems in the infant-parent mutual attachment process need to be individually addressed, depending upon the specific case. The question of how long therapeutic interventions are continued is strongly tied to the severity of the disturbance and the specifics of exacerbating or ameliorating factors. The question of flexibility in the number of sessions per month, in the format of the intervention within each session, and in the variety of techniques used is also addressed.

In discussing the length of treatment for "average" mothers, D. Stern (personal communication, August 1989) stated that interventions, directed at the problems in mother-infant interactions that are detrimental to the attachment process, are typically brief. Several sessions may suffice. I have also had the experience that this is the case for some mothers, those who are non-psychotic.

For instance, Joyce, who had always been a functioning member of society, was married, held a responsible, complex job, and had a small child who was very well adjusted and bright, provides an example of short-term dyadic psychotherapy treatment. Joyce was presently in a reactive state of anxiety due to illness in her husband, which had an enormous negative economic impact upon them. Among other things, it required them to move back to her parents' house.

This was experienced as highly stressful by Joyce. She then resented the birth of her new baby, which coincided with this setback. Joyce, a highly controlled person, was not able to vent or otherwise deal with her negative feelings. She became constricted in her interactions with her new baby, avoiding eye contact, and generally having minimal contact with her. At the same time, she denied her negative feelings and was starting to project them onto the new baby. The baby, in turn, was reacting progressively less to her mother. The baby had developed gaze aversion and, though a robust baby, was starting to lose interest in her surroundings, including food. She was developing a *failure-to-thrive* syndrome. This mother and infant, indeed, required only two dyadic sessions, intermingled with three individual sessions for the mother alone.

With this short-term dyadic psychotherapy, there was a dramatic change in their interactions. The mother's negative behavior changed to positive, which enabled the infant to thrive and continue her development on course. The mother had been able to gain some limited insight into her intrapsychic problems, as well as some insight in relation to her feelings about her husband, consequently improving her interactions with him.

Through the dyadic psychotherapy, she had also been able to elicit positive emotional responsivity from her baby, and was helped to be able to feel good about this, as well as to appreciate her own ability to elicit these reactions contingently. Attachment had been largely lacking. To the extent to which it had been present, it had been developing in a negative direction. Now attachment proceeded in a positive vein. Both mother and infant were able to take joy in each other's interactions.

In this example, it can be seen that when there are early attachment problems in the process of developing, brief intervention may suffice in the case of the "normal" parent. In many instances, this is the case for the neurotic parent as well. However, when severe emotional problems exist, such as in psychosis, the mother is in need of a sustained psycho-therapeutic relationship.

The advent of the birth of a new baby, and its anticipation, do provide a special opportunity for renewal and change. The woman is more highly motivated at this time: she wants to be a good mother and wants her child to have a chance in life. At some level of awareness, she knows that this is not easy for her, although she may not be able to verbalize this clearly. The parent is amenable to intervention, if there is a hope that it will help her baby. Furthermore, she is in a more dependent emotional state at this time, which consequently adds to her tendency to accept therapeutic contact.

There are other advantages to this moment of opportunity for engaging the mother therapeutically, ranging from the "normal" to the psychotic woman. At the extreme of the spectrum, many psychotics are so constricted, defended, or depressed that they are essentially unable to engage in verbal interactions. Much of the substance of the dyadic psychotherapy is related to the behavioral interactions between mother and infant; it is non-verbal. Thus therapeutic interventions do not require verbalizations on the part of the patient and can proceed in a natural flow despite this lack. In fact, typically, in the initial phases of therapy, these mothers tend to be minimally reactive, not only to the baby but also in general, including to the therapist.

These parents tend to sit quietly with the baby over their lap, looking into space ("log effect"). As the therapeutic process continues, the patient feels more comfortable and becomes somewhat more communicative. Consequently, there tends to be more verbal production by patients in this second phase of therapy. Since the severely disturbed patient has many intrapsychic issues, and since most are at multi-risk with many difficult interpersonal, environmental, economic, educational, and vocational problems, it is found that these other risk areas also demand attention.

Frequently, as the mother-infant attachment process improves, the mother's self-image and feeling of competency also improve. She consequently will tend to broaden her vistas and seek to improve herself in other areas of her life. She will make or improve social contacts, aspire to improved economic circumstances, and may strive for vocational training and for work. Therefore, although the primary goal of dyadic psychotherapy is the prevention of psychopathology in the infant, the mother typically makes gains in her adjustment. (The bipolar tends not to benefit greatly, quickly enough, because of the intransigence of her conviction of her own worthlessness and consequent tendency to continue to cycle through severe mood changes.)

It is also because of the severity of the disturbance that the need for continued therapeutic interventions persists. The child's positive development through the formative years is needed as a base for continued adequate emotional development. In particular, the psychotic mother will need the availability of continued psychotherapy, guidance, and support through this time. Developmental hurdles are particularly difficult. The child's self-assertiveness and striving for independence are easily experienced as a threat by the mother. The availability of the therapist is paramount for these mothers. Generally about two years of dyadic psychotherapy is needed.

Flexibility within the therapy process is also important, both in the number of sessions per month and in the format of the intervention within the sessions. It may be that a mother will need to continue after the intensive phase is completed, to have sessions infrequently, or perhaps on an as-needed basis. Within the session, it is always necessary to be open to the mother's pressing issues. Therefore, though a given dyadic psychotherapy session is focused on attachment issues between mother and infant, some of the content may center around the mother's fears, anxieties, and symptoms. The infant, during these discussions, recedes to the background of the sessions. In so doing, the mother also learns that the baby has the strength to not be the constant focus of attention, and is able to occupy itself. At the same time the baby is never out of the mother's and therapist's awareness; if attention is demanded or required, the baby is attended to. If the mother does not spontaneously do so, and move to provide what the baby needs, the therapist focuses attention on the baby and makes sure that the mother provides what is needed. A variety of techniques are used in doing this, ranging from least intrusive and least imperative to molding and directives.

Sometimes an opportunity offers itself to provide an incisive interpretation of the mother's psychodynamics. Such an opportunity should never be lost. The dyadic psychotherapist has a deep and long-term relationship with the patient. Although she may not typically discuss deeply dynamic issues, there is nevertheless a strong therapeutic alliance with the therapist. Consequently, the mother may at times suddenly mention something that has great significance in her psychopathology. Such incisions into the psychopathology, under these circumstances, have proved highly effective in improving the anxiety level and adjustment of the patient from that point forward.

The length of dyadic psychotherapy for psychotic mothers and their infants is typically at least two years of intensive (an hour or more per week) intervention, with continued, less frequent contact after that. It can span the period from pregnancy through the fourth year of life of the infant. Should the child still have emotional problems at that point, an appropriate additional individual treatment plan will still be needed. Typically, we find that if there has been no neurological or other damage to the child, he/she will be developing adequately and with no massive emotional problems by this time. The mother may well need to continue to receive therapeutic and/or case management services.

9

Positive Outcomes of Dyadic Psychotherapy

What are some positive outcomes of dyadic psychotherapy? Outcomes vary. Two cases with diametrically opposite outcomes may both be considered positive depending on the case characteristics. Increased positive infant-parent attachment, as well as emotional acceptance of infant-parent separation, can each be positive outcomes, depending on the case.

What is truly exciting in this work is this writer's discovery that even in the very worst case scenarios of severely psychotic and "underclass" mothers, and even in the face of the absolutely worst possible socioeconomic and cultural factors, with dyadic psychotherapy there is still significant evidence for hope in a variety of positive outcomes. There is significant evidence that intervention prevents later psychopathology and allows for an adequate start in life during the baby's early developmental years.

How effective is dyadic psychotherapy? Based on the results of the clinical interventions, even in the very worst case scenarios, those of severely disturbed and psychotic mothers, there are positive outcomes.

ENHANCED ATTACHMENT

There are various outcomes of dyadic psychotherapy which can be considered positive. The most obvious is when mother and infant attach well, and when the father is also an integral, attached part of the family.

For instance, Laura, age twenty, has a history of psychiatric hospitalizations since childhood. She withdrew emotionally during pregnancy and was rehospitalized during the puerperium. She was referred for dyadic psychotherapy at this time. The interventions involved Jacob, the father of the baby. For a period of time Jacob performed the maternal functions, and he attached to the infant, Cyril. Gradually the mother assumed the maternal functions. As she improved and left in-patient services, Jacob resumed his breadwinning functions. Through psychotherapeutic interventions, he was helped to maintain the existing attachment and transform it into protective functions for his family.

Both parents were helped to focus on Cyril's development. In so doing, they were able to learn to understand their baby's needs, to recognize his developmental milestones, and to enjoy his accomplishments. The mother's psychotic discomfort was alleviated. They learned to respect the infant's growth and to allow him to determine his own interests, both when he was being fed and when he was at play. The mother was helped to become less intrusive, with the help of the father, who moderated the mother-infant interactions. The infant was acquiring a longer attention span, persistence, and goal orientation. Both parents protected the infant from what they perceived as a disruptive external world. They took pride in their accomplishments as parents, and they themselves changed as a result of having assumed their respective parenting roles.

ACCEPTANCE OF SEPARATION

There is another possible outcome that can be desirable: when a mother who is not capable of mothering her infant, due to her extremely debilitating psychosis, is finally able to acknowledge this inability. In dyadic psychotherapy, she comes to accept this on her own, through her interactions with the infant and in terms of the child's development.

For instance, the behavior of Melinda, age thirty-two, had deteriorated steadily over the eight years prior to her present hospitalization. Although hospitalized twice during these eight years, her diagnosis was still inaccurate, and she was not treated effectively. Her mental state deteriorated steadily. She lost her job, then her marriage, and then custody of her oldest child. Her home was auctioned off. Finally, she became homeless and pregnant. At this time she was referred for treatment, following a violent incident. She was deeply damaged and devoid of environmental supports. She was nevertheless able to come to terms with the fact that she would not be able to reconstruct herself and her world in time for her child's development, and therefore the best alternative open to her was to relinquish the child. The success of the therapy, in this case, was measured and evidenced in her ability to make this difficult decision, and thereby to begin to heal. After this decision, which she felt was in the best interests of her child, the work of helping her to "mourn" for her lost infant was accomplished in the therapy. This creative woman decided to write biannual letters to her child in which she informed him about her deteriorating illness and her work of reconstruction of herself, so that when he grew up he would be proud of his mother's example. She deposited the letters with the adopting agency, to be opened at the adoptive parents' discretion, at an age at which he would be able to understand them. In this case, the infant was also the stimulator of the mother's wish to grow and develop, so that he would not need to be ashamed of her.

OTHER OUTCOMES

There are many outcomes that fall between the two previous examples of attachment and separation. These occur when the mother and the child are not in the traditional nuclear family and when the mother relinquishes the child for adoption. In most instances, the mother has no support or, at best, inconsistent support from the infant's father; the extended family is either not supportive or is inconsistently supportive; and/or the primary caretaker is someone other than the mother (another family member or foster parent). In these instances, the desirable outcome also varies. It may be, for example that the mother is gradually able to become more active or more emotionally contributory to the caretaking of the infant, or that the mother can gradually take over the primary care of the infant, with a good deal of agency support. When this outcome occurs, previous support people frequently resurface, or the mother herself is able to develop new relationships which offer relief from her emotional isolation, as well as the emotional isolation of the child.

One example is of a mother, Elly, who had been severely depressed for two years prior to being referred. Before her breakdown she had been able to be productive in her life. She had two children, a three-year-old, Gigi, and a one-and-a-half-year-old, Don. She had been hospitalized soon after Don's birth, and thus they had never been attached to each other. In fact Don did not remember his mother. Gigi did remember her, but was highly apprehensive with Elly at first encounter, actually having some negative reactions to her. Through weekly dyadic psychotherapy with each of the children over a period of a year, the children and the mother gradually attached to each other. Though highly reluctant to communicate her feelings verbally, the mother was able to work through her fears and her feelings of ineptitude and guilt about having abandoned the children. She was able to change her negative pattern of interactions to positive patterns and to react empathically to the children. Her improvement also brought with it more mutual acceptance in relation to her family, as well as the development of new relationships. Further, aspiring to re-enter the work world, Elly was able to allow room in this agenda for establishing a home with her children. This was accomplished only with a good deal of agency intervention in obtaining a home and school/day care for the children. With help, she has been able to move forward in all areas of her life.

Another example is of a mother, Pat, who was a revolving-door patient and whose family was replete with psychotic relatives. Pat started in therapy during the latter part of her pregnancy. She was able, as a consequence, to survive parturition without further decompensation. Furthermore, she was able to be the primary caretaker of the child, Tom, for his first two and a half years. Tom developed well in all areas, though he weighed only four pounds at birth. Pat was able to experience joy and satisfaction in her attachment with Tom, and Tom was playful and emotionally well developed. Under constant inner and environmental pressure, Pat allowed Tom to be taken away by a relative at two and a half years of age. Although she wanted to keep him, she was ambivalent, feeling that Tom would have a better life with the relative. Pat is satisfied in that she gave him a firm foundation in his early formative years and that he is continuing to do well. She feels that she was the real, that is, the psychological, mother to Tom, in contrast to her relationship to her previous children, and she takes great satisfaction in this. She has not felt the need to have another baby, as is the typical scenario without dyadic psychotherapy, because she had experienced a true relatedness with Tom.

OUTLOOK

Throughout this work, based on the author's findings, there is a much more optimistic stance about what is possible and what is preventable for at-risk children, even when due to psychotic mothering. Fish (1984), in her work, concluded that early interventions might be developed to arrest, prevent, or compensate for various deficits in high-risk infants which become evident prior to two years of age. The present writer reports that it is indeed possible to do so. With dyadic psychotherapy it is possible to intervene in order to change the trend that leads to the formation of psychopathology, through concerted and focused psychotherapeutic efforts, coupled with the engagement of environmental supports. With appropriate dyadic psychotherapy intervention, it is possible to help the disturbed mother—and also father and significant others—sufficiently to resolve the fears and conflicts of relating with the infant to allow them to act in the best interests of the child. Dyadic psychotherapy intervention promotes the at-risk child's experience of "good-enough" mothering. This is done in order for the child to gain the basic developmental foundations to allow for an adequate start in life during the vitally important early developmental years.

10

Other Types of Cases That Benefit from Dyadic Psychotherapy

Previous chapters have taken the worst psychopathology in the mother as the risk factor for the child. Other scenarios are briefly touched upon in this chapter: the drug addict, those with characterological problems, the teen parent, the single parent, and the "normal" parent.

ADDICTION

Work with mothers who are in treatment for their drug addiction has shown that the basic dyadic psychotherapy approach outlined in the previous chapters is applicable for these mothers, as well. Their behavior with their infants varies according to their diagnoses, beyond their drug addiction, and thus the interventions will vary accordingly.

Typically there are complicating factors in their lives related to the addiction, such as their "significant other" male friend. He is, on the average, a non-emotionally supportive person, who himself has severe character problems, and consequently misuses the woman. Therefore, attention to this relationship is frequently an important part of the intervention. This requires the woman to gain a stronger self-image and some understanding of the psychodynamics of staying in a destructive relationship. This is important for the well-being of both the mother and the baby.

These psychodynamics tend to stem from abusive treatment sustained by the mother in her early developmental years. In many cases, she has been the victim of sexual abuse. What remains within her is her fear, anger, and rage, as well as her peculiar way of interpreting herself and the world around her.

Most substance abusers, similar to all other mothers, want their children to have a good life. When they are driven by their addiction, however, the addiction is primary. They are therefore unable to give priority to the needs of their child and will neglect and/or abuse the child, or allow others to do so.

Such mothers need to be in treatment, concomitantly, for their substance abuse, in order to be able to benefit from dyadic psychotherapy. The child needs to be protected. This has been found to work successfully on an outpatient basis, however, with a good deal of intensive and varied interventions.

CHARACTER PROBLEMS

The predominant, relevant, central trait of people with severe characterological problems is their lack of empathy for others. They have made their adjustment to the world in centering all their efforts on self-gratification, though never able to fill the internal narcissistic void.

The attachment of such a mother to her child can be bolstered to the extent that she can be helped to react empathetically to him/her. Also, to the extent that the mother can thereby experience attachment to the child, she will also gain a sense of existence herself. This, in turn, helps her to interact more empathetically with her baby. Since motherhood is a centrally important part of the identity of most women (those who want children), the sense of being a "good" mother is a highly significant growth factor in the life cycle development of the woman. It consequently tends to strengthen the mother's sense of self and to enhance her self-concept. In addition to the benefit to the mother, this strengthening benefits her relationship with her child, as well as the child's development.

TEEN PARENT

In our culture, the teenager has certain tasks to accomplish. These include completing her education in order to enable her to deal with our extremely competitive society, and to develop emotionally to the point of being emotionally self-sufficient, at least to a large extent.

If this has not been accomplished, the teen feels cheated if she is not allowed to continue on this course. Furthermore, she is not ready to take on a primarily nurturing role demanded by being a parent (versus the role of being nurtured, in being a child). Consequently, being a teen parent is intrinsically problematic.

Beyond that, it appears that most teen parents have vague and unrealistic expectations of the partner and of the baby. They are emotionally hurt when these expectations are not realized. In fact, in most cases the father of the baby exits the romantic relationship either prior to or soon after the birth of the baby. The infant, contrary to expectation, does not immediately supply love, but rather is a demanding bundle of needs. The teen mother is disappointed. Her ability to care for the infant effectively and to develop a positive attachment is dependent on her own emotional developmental level and the soundness of her psychological armamentarium. She can be helped to strengthen her positive attachment to her infant, both directly in the dyadic psychotherapy and indirectly by aiding her to seek the help she needs in caring for her infant.

SINGLE PARENT

Parenting is a draining task. Both the infant and the child require constant monitoring and care. There is little or no respite. When extended families live together, there is the possibility that others will be available to share in the care of the child. In our society it is frequently the case that the nuclear family lives alone. When this family is constituted of only one adult, the entire burden falls on her. The single parent must arrange for some kind of respite care in order to have any time for herself. Even then, the emotional burden of caring for the child remains exclusively hers.

Again, the effectiveness of her mothering will depend on her level of emotional development and psychological wholeness. However, any problems will be magnified because the child has only her to relate to. It is therefore advisable to set the interaction between mother and child on a good course from the beginning by helping her to develop a positive empathic attachment. When this happens, there is a sense of relatedness and joy, a deep sense of satisfaction, which overshadows the arduousness of the task of caring for one's child.

"NORMAL"

The "normal" parents are those without major impediments in their emotional/psychological makeup. They may have some degree of any, or a combination of, problems previously discussed, which impinge on their manner of relating to their children.

Even for "normal" parents, who generally have inconsequential or minor problems within themselves, there can be times when they find themselves under inordinate stress through the vicissitudes of living in our complex and difficult world. Should the timing of this stress coincide with the advent of a new baby, there may be consequences to the quality of care. If the parent finds him/herself emotionally spent by the stress, or if minor psychopathology is exacerbated by it, there is the possibility of problems for the child. In these circumstances, dyadic psychotherapy may be indicated. The focus would, as usual, be on the attachment process/relationship, but also on the relief of the experienced stress and on clarification of unrealistic fantasies and attributions. In this kind of case, the intervention may be very brief. Several sessions may suffice. The impact of the brief intervention may, however, be monumental in terms of the wholesome development of the infant, now being free of interferences with the positive attachment process with his/her parent(s).

11

Conclusions

Most parents are able to bring up their children adequately, so that they are able to take their place as productive members of society. Most are able to meet their children's basic and emotional needs. Most are able to provide food and shelter, education, and love to their children in sufficient amounts, quality, and distribution in time to enable the child to thrive and develop. Amazingly the deepest, most gratifying, and sustaining phenomenon develops between people; it is called attachment. The first and strongest attachment develops during infancy, with the primary caretaker(s). In order for a strong, positive attachment to develop, certain ingredients need to be present. In the average course of events, for normal dyads, these ingredients are taken as a matter of course. It is when the ingredients are lacking, insufficient, or inappropriate that their very presence is noted; that is what this book has devoted itself to exploring.

In normal circumstances, the mother falls in love with her baby, and the baby falls in love with the mother. This happens when they are open to receiving the sensory/perceptual input from each other and they are not blocked from taking pleasure from this. That is, the mother looks into the baby's eyes; the baby looks at the mother. They gaze at each other. The baby smiles; the mother smiles. The mother feels the baby snuggled in her arms; the baby reciprocates the molding. The baby gurgles and coos; the mother "talks" to the baby. There is a reciprocity of perceptual and motor interplay which is highly satisfying and gives tremendous pleasure to both. These are the ingredients for the development of attachment between them. A strong positive attachment allows the infant to develop emotion-ally and later to develop wholesome attachments to others. The child is thereby able to navigate through life without major emotional disasters (if the seas are not excessively rough). Sometimes, as described here, dyadic psychotherapy may be helpful to get through the more "normal," or neurotic, parent/infant rough spots.

However, when there are problems with the essential ingredients for attachment, living one's life is problematic. This book has dealt with some of the most serious hurdles in attachment. Psychoses interfere with func-tioning in general. The focus here has been on interferences in the mother/infant interactions and on psychotherapeutic interventions to deal with these.

One characteristic all mothers appear to have in common is that they want a good life for their child. Even the most dysfunctional have this idea. This motivation allows for therapeutic intervention where pre-viously it may have been more difficult. It allows for an early opportunity to offer the mother the development of a degree of emotional clarity with which to interact with and regard her child. Sometimes this results in a realization on the part of the mother that she will not be able to function adequately enough in time for her child. In some cases, she can then work, in the interests of her child, toward relinquishing it. In other cases the mother may be helped to interact with her baby in an increasingly adequate and satisfying manner, allowing the child to develop sufficiently well emotionally.

Typically the mother is helped to have a sense of having tried her best at mothering, that is, of being a good mother to her child. She may also have made some gains in terms of her own adjustment. The child will have been helped to develop a positive sense of self and a sense of having the ability to cope with life. The child will have been spared the worst obstacles to adequate emotional development. The attempt is to effect this, whether the child is with other caretakers or remains in the care of the mother. The next generation need not carry the burdens of its parents.

Appendix A

Psychodiagnostic Differences in Auditory and Vestibular Stimulation in Mothering

Prior to providing clinical services to mothers and infants, questions concerning mother-infant interactions were addressed in a study. The study, which is abstracted here, was designed to explore specific differences in mothers' stimulation of their infants according to diagnosis (Gochman and Aisenstein, 1985). The study found that there were distinct differences which reflected diagnostic differences in a very significant manner. The next step was to elaborate a therapeutic intervention for mothers that would benefit the emotional development of their infants.

We know that sensory stimulation in the various modalities has importance to people of all ages for their general functioning. Animal and human studies indicate the critical importance of neonates' experiences in the first months of life for both physical and psychological development. Deprived of early stimulation, infants are at risk for cognitive delays and delays in emotional development (Brossard and Decarie, 1968; Casler, 1965; Wright, 1971; Yarrow, Rubenstein, and Pedersen, 1975).

One of the sensory areas that has been given attention is the area of vestibular stimulation (Bender, 1956; Korner, 1972; Ornitz, 1970; Spitz, 1965). We also know from observation that vestibular stimulation is important in soothing babies, such as in gently rocking them. Not all parents are the same in how they handle their babies; there are substantial individual differences (Musick, Clark, Cohler, and Dincin, 1979). Some parents provide very little verbal or vestibular stimulation to their infants and children. When this lack is extreme, resultant difficulties may emerge in the children's general development and in the language area (Lennenberg, 1976; Provence and Lipton, 1962; Yarrow, 1961). Mothers who talk more to their infants tend to have infants who vocalize more (Haugan and McIntire, 1972). There seem to be differences between mothers of various psychodiagnostic categories in how they interact with their infants, and consequently how they impact in these two areas of stimulation; schizophrenic women provide less vestibular stimulation and vocalize less with their infants than normal mothers (Grunebaum, Weiss, Cohler, Hartman, and Gallant, 1975; Korner, 1972; Sobel, 1961). In general, children of disturbed mothers are at risk, in their development, for a broad range of psychopathology, particularly children of schizophrenic mothers (Garmezy and Streitman, 1974; Sameroff, 1975; Silverton, Finello, and Mednick, 1983; Watt, Anthony, Wynne, and Rolf, 1984).

The first task for the study was to gather participants. They were recruited in gynecology clinics of the child health clinics of a large metropolitan city. Participants were similar across diagnostic categories in all of the socioeconomic, social, and cultural factors. The Schachter Scale (Schachter, 1970; Schachter, Kerr, Lachine, and Faer, 1975; Wright, 1971) was used as a screening instrument, during the last trimester of pregnancy, to gather potential participants. All the women were functioning in the community, adapting at various levels of reality. Participants were subsequently tested on the Rorschach Inkblot Test when their babies were two months old. Some were found, both on the Schachter Scale and on the Rorschach Inkblot Test, to evidence an underlying schizophrenic process. They were classified on the DSM III (American Psychiatric Association, 1980) as having a schizoid personality disorder, or paranoid personality disorder. Those with low psychopathology were considered "normal" and were used for comparison purposes.

One overall question was which specific psychodiagnostic groups to observe in order to contrast infant stimulation. Clinically, paranoid schizophrenics tend more to maintain their level of integration and functioning when they are contrasted to other types of schizophrenics. They were divided accordingly into paranoid and non-paranoid participants.

Mothers with their infants were seen in a series of three weekly observation sessions starting when the infant was one month old. These sessions were videotaped. They were then scored for the presence or absence of vestibular and auditory stimulation, for five-second intervals.

Vestibular stimulation was considered to be taking place if the baby's head (body) position was changed by the mother. Auditory stimulation was considered to be taking place if the mother made sounds (talked, sang, etc.) which could be heard by the baby. The sessions were partly with the mother and baby alone in the room, and part of the time an observer was present in the room with them.

It was found that those mothers with paranoid personality disorders tend to stimulate their infants more than "normal" mothers and than non-paranoid mothers with schizoid personality disorders. The latter tend to stimulate their infants somewhat less than "normal" mothers. This is so for both vestibular and auditory stimulation. These differences were more pronounced when the mother and infant were alone than when the observer was in the same room.

It is as though the mothers with paranoid personality disorders are super-stimulators, while the non-paranoid mothers with schizoid personality disorders are under-stimulators. The importance of the distinction between non-paranoid and paranoid mothers is highlighted. It has particular importance in terms of understanding potential differences in the development of their children, as well as in the planning of interventions.

The implication of these findings is that intervention for non-paranoid mothers (with schizoid personality disorders) and their infants tend to require an attempt to increase stimulation for the infants, while interventions for paranoid (personality disordered) mothers would tend to require other goals, perhaps to lessen intrusive over-stimulation.

Appendix B

A Comparison of Two Normal Mothers' Mothering

In the course of doing the study "High-Risk Stimulation," normal mothers were seen as control subjects. Two of these mothers offered an interesting comparison in that they each brought a second child, a toddler, to some sessions. This created a more complex situation in which observation of the mothering style could be compared. The similarities and differences between these mothers are presented and are related to broad differences in personality structure.

Two "normal" mothers brought their one-month-old infants for participation in the Mother and Infant research project. These two mothers had a good deal in common but were highly divergent in their behaviors with their infants. They were seen for observation sessions, the purpose of which was to obtain taped sessions of mother-infant interactions for a broader study (Gochman and Aisenstein, 1985). Each of these mothers brought the next oldest sibling, a toddler, to a session, allowing for observations of the triad.

It could be hypothesized that an additional child being present in the situation would tend to stimulate the mother, and that this in turn would activate her, resulting in increased stimulation of her infant. The behavior of these two mothers, however, was quite divergent in this regard. One mother, A. J., was one of the highest stimulators of the sample, while the other mother, E. P., was the lowest stimulator, by a wide margin, in one modality (vestibular) and within the medium range in another (auditory stimulation).

VIGNETTES OF THE TWO MOTHERS

Both mothers are low-socioeconomic level, inner-city black women. Both were brought up in a nuclear family household where mother and father were married and where the mother was the primary caretaker of the children. Both have maintained a long-term relationship with the father of their baby, and these fathers take responsibility for the children and help in their support. Both fathers are employed. Both mothers are considered normal in psychiatric interview and exhibit no gross pathology in psychological testing. Neither mother has a drug or alcohol abuse problem. Both mothers have more than one older child. They both had a pleasant pregnancy and gave birth uneventfully.

Anne was an only child. She is thirty-four years old. She completed twelve years of schooling. Her first sexual experience was at eighteen years. She had two other children, two- and nine-year-old boys, in addition to the infant, another boy. She lives with her parents. She does not smoke or drink. She has known the father of the baby for about four years. He is forty-three years old, is employed, lives nearby, and helps with material needs. Her mother helps with the baby. She has plans to return to her job as a secretary in the school system.

Edith was the youngest of six siblings, four brothers and two sisters. She is twenty-four years old. She completed ten years of schooling. She drinks some beer and smokes. Her first sexual experience was at fifteen years of age. She has three other children, an eight-year-old boy, a six-year-old boy, and a one-and-a-half-year-old girl, in addition to the infant, a girl. She lives with her husband and children, a nuclear family. Her husband also completed ten years of schooling. She has known him since she was thirteen years old. He is now twenty-six years old, is employed, and helps with chores and with the children when he gets home from work. She has been employed as a telephone operator; however, her plans are to return to school.

Despite these similarities between the mothers, striking differences exist between them, in both their personalities and their behavior with their children. Though both are in the normal range, personality differences are reflected on psychological testing. For Anne, the total number of responses for the Rorschach test is fourteen, while for Edith, it is nine. Anne rejects no cards, while Edith rejects three cards. Anne is able to give a color response, while Edith is not. Anne gives a balance of human movement and animal movement responses; Edith has no human movement responses and only one animal movement response (form responses predominate for her). The total number of determinants used by Anne is five, versus two by Edith. In general, the difference points to a broader response repertoire, a somewhat more expansive, less constricted personality, and a higher energy level on the part of Anne.

The difference is clearly reflected in the dyad observations. Anne is one of the highest stimulators of her infant in comparison to other mothers in both modalities measured in this study, auditory and vestibular. On the other hand, Edith is the lowest vestibular stimulator, and only a medium stimulator in the auditory realm.

Comparison of the triad sessions yields further contrasts. In these situations the mothers have an additional child present, a toddler. This complicates the interactional situation and interestingly highlights differences. Anne is very much relaxed. She interacts easily with both her infant and her toddler simultaneously. She involves the toddler in activities with the baby, and casually teaches her toddler, simultaneously, parts of the body of the toy dog. She talks to and plays with the infant pleasantly.

In contrast, Edith has less success in coordinating herself with her two children. She plays with her infant, but at the expense of the toddler, who consequently indulges in a variety of attention-seeking behaviors; he "accidentally" spills some milk, leaves the room, starts to answer the phone, and climbs onto a high changing table, putting himself in danger. At one point the toddler tries to get mother's attention directly. Annoyed, she hits him lightly on his hands; the toddler makes a fist, as though to fight. At another point the mother says to her toddler that she will read a children's book to him, which she proceeds to read to herself only. In general, there are long periods of silence, with the mother not interacting with either child.

It is clear that the differences in the mother's own personalities are reflected in their levels of stimulation of their infants and in their interactions with their infants and toddlers. Clearly, the more constricted mother stimulates her infant less than the mother with a richer repertoire of psychological responsivity. The more constricted mother's lacks are less clear in the dyad situation, but are highlighted as the complexity of the situation increases when her toddler is also present; she is unable to integrate easily the handling of both children simultaneously. Attention-seeking behaviors emerge on the part of the toddler, which are handled punitively by the mother. These in turn are followed by hostile reactions on the part of the toddler. Thereby a negative interactive cycle proceeds to emerge.

The mother with the larger response repertoire, on the other hand, has no difficulty integrating both the infant and toddler into mutual interactions. There are no acting-out behaviors on the part of the toddler, nor negative cycling interactions. Instead there is an ease and comfort in the interactions.

The comparisons of these two "normal" mothers demonstrates the relationship between a mother's own personality and her behavior vis-à-vis her one-month-old infant. It is clear that the behavior of the mother is directly linked to personality structure, and expressed in a more pronounced manner when the situation the mother finds herself in is more complex. Implications of this study include:

1. Mothers with a constricted response repertoire function less well in a more complex situation. Therefore, they would do well to have help from support people in bringing up their child(ren). The implied need for this would tend to increase geometrically with increased complexities, such as the presence of more children.

2. Children seek the mother's attention. If they are unable to obtain it in a relaxed, acceptable fashion, they will start to develop less acceptable ways. That is, they will pragmatically use whatever works in getting that attention. This tends to be behavior referred to as "acting-out" behavior. The unacceptability of that behavior tends to cycle a punitive reaction in the mother, which in turn engenders hostility in the child. The result is then further acting out, which now has an additional motivation and tends to continue the cycle of negative interactions.

The utility of increasing the response repertoire of the mother, as a preventive measure, in relation to the negative cycling between mother and child, is desirable.

Appendix C

Three Clinical Bylines

In the course of many years of providing clinical interventions to mothers and infants, many interesting observations have been made. Presented here are three memorable observations, each of which has far-reaching implications for clinical understanding of behavior and interventions for mothers and infants.

"An Infant's Panic" is an abstract of a study (Gochman, 1989b) which describes the ability of the infant to sense danger from negative symptoms. "The Psychodynamic Purposiveness of a Kidnapping" is an abstract (Gochman, 1989a) illustrating a mother's unconscious process that serves in the best interests of her child. "Abandonment of the Institutional Stare in a Toddler" describes the high efficiency of dyadic psychotherapy in achieving positive results within several sessions.

AN INFANT'S PANIC

An infant cries when distressed, when its integrity is threatened. This may be due to physical discomfort and/or noxious threats. In order to perceive threat, a degree of sensory, cognitive, and emotional integration is required. The anticipation of threat to integrity is anxiety. According to Horner (1980), anxiety emerges with any perceived threat to the integrity of the self; and for Brossard (1974), it is in terms of the ego's reactions to or anticipation of danger. Anxiety requires the perception of danger (Slucking, 1964; Bird, 1980). To exhibit "stranger anxiety" the infant must have learned to differentiate the familiar (mother) from the non-familiar person (stranger). The mothering person provides the key to understanding anxiety (Schecter, 1980). When there is secure attachment, an absence of the mothering person is seen as a threat by the infant. When positive attachment is lacking, stranger anxiety is absent or is exhibited in a distorted manner. Peculiar infant behavior has been observed (between three and eighteen months) to extreme danger and deprivation, which can be manifested in early defenses of "avoidance," "freezing," and "fighting" (Fraiberg, 1982). "Signal anxiety" (Horner, 1980) can develop with re-peated stressful stimuli. It remains unclear what specific stimuli the infant uses to sense danger.

Generally, when infants have displayed panic and defensive behaviors, this has been attributed to a history of noxious caretaking or to stranger anxiety. The totality of prior interactions between the mother and infant are typically not known. When all interactions between a given mother and infant have been observed directly, it is of great interest.

In this case, observations were made on a mother (and infant) who had been incarcerated during her pregnancy and postpartum. During the index (observation) session the baby was seven months old. The mother and baby had had six sessions over the seven-month period, always with the therapist (or other staff) present. She had never been alone with the baby. On observation, the child had not yet developed stranger anxiety.

The mother had attacked a relative with a knife. She had been hospital-ized for two years with a diagnosis of schizophrenia. She was extremely uncommunicative and unresponsive to all around her, including the thera-pist, on the day of the index session.

Before encountering her mother, the baby was animated, happy and interactive; this included smiling, eye contact, and waving to other strangers while alone with the therapist. The baby became glum at seeing her mother. When handed to the mother she turned back to the therapist with panic. She cried unrelentingly while held by the mother. After a half hour of active therapeutic intervention, the infant was soothed, though still teary-eyed.

During the index session the mother had an impassive mask-like ex-pression on her face and was inactive. She did hold the baby gently and was pleased to see her. There was nothing overtly noxious in her treatment, facial expression, or manner of holding the baby. At the end of the session the baby readily separated from her mother and subsequently regained her cheerfulness.

During the next session the mother was less depressed, in better spirits, and more natural with her baby. The baby did not cry, though she was still glum in the presence of her mother.

During the index session the infant had reacted to her mother as though she had been abused by her. In fact, she had not been abused. Instead, the baby was apparently reacting to a particular configuration of stimuli emanating from the mother. These may have included an impassive appearance, lack of soothing behavior, lack of joy, and rigidity in the face and body. The infant seems to have utilized these cues and reacted with panic, as though she was afraid of suffering at the hands of this mother.

This case points to the complexity of anxiety in the developing infant. The infant perceived subtle cues from the mother which served to signal real danger. These cues did not include overtly noxious or punitive handling. The anxiety was specific to one person (the mother), as distinct from her reaction to others. The anxiety was not stranger anxiety, nor a result of either physical discomfort or unmet needs, or repeated stressful stimuli. The anxiety was specific to subtle cues, probably in the facial expression of the mother (or lack of facial expression), which the infant experienced as a threat to herself.

By implication, it may be that in cases where abuse develops, this interaction typifies the germinal phases. The mother's impassive handling of the child leads to the child's negative reaction to the mother, which the mother cannot tolerate, and which then creates a negative cycling in their interaction pattern. Abuse may easily become an end product of such a pattern. When a primary caretaker has this kind of impact on the child the infant will make an adjustment to the situation, which constitutes the eventual development of defenses or symptoms of psychopathology.

THE PSYCHODYNAMIC PURPOSIVENESS OF A KIDNAPPING

Her three-year-old son was in foster care. With reunification as the objective, the biological mother and her son were seen in dyadic psychotherapy. She gradually came to recognize that her child was doing well in his foster home. They wanted to adopt him. The mother slowly came to the decision, with some pain, that it would be best for him and would give him a "good life." Though she denied it, she remained conflicted, in that her mother was opposed. Her giving up her son would threaten her symbiotic relationship with her mother; she had a strong need for her mother's approval. After this decision the mother missed a series of sessions. She then changed her mind about allowing her son to be adopted. When she reappeared she was uncommunicative, then seized the moment, grabbed her son, and ran away with him, kidnapping him. The foster mother and therapist overtook her. She relinquished the child readily, and appeared to be calm and satisfied.

Although initially very much upset, after a week, the child was calm about the incident. In fact, he appeared to have resolved his conflicts about his mother, solidified his integration into the foster family, and had improved his adjustment. He abandoned his nightmares, persistent phobias, and bedwetting.

The child's history included abuse by his grandmother and neglect by his schizoaffective, alcoholic, mother. They had at times been homeless, living on the street and in abandoned buildings, where there had been an incident of severe abuse by other children.

Why did this kidnapping attempt fail? This bright young woman could have done it more effectively. Though attached to her son, this mother had therapeutically worked through a decision to allow him to be adopted so that he could have "a good life," despite her pain in so doing. Furthermore, her symbiotic relationship with her mother was now in jeopardy. The kidnapping served as a solution. She felt that this absolved her in her mother's eyes from the blame of giving her son up. Her relationship with her mother could now continue, and she could maintain her mother's emotional support. Her son was freed from his conflicts about giving her up, in that it placed her in the "bad mother" role and allowed him to see his foster mother as the "good mother." She had taken a chance. She tried the kidnapping with the unconscious wish *not to succeed*. The mother's unconscious worked to free her child of conflict and herself from guilt. What she wanted was a "good life" for her child.

ABANDONMENT OF THE INSTITUTIONAL STARE IN A TODDLER

Two-year-old Betsy was brought to the session by a nurse from the orphanage. The child bore an institutional stare. She was timid, constricted, playing carefully with few toys, not vocalizing, and was hypersensitive to even the slightest sounds. The wide-open, hypervigilant eyes predominated her emotionless face.

Her mother, Mrs. A, had been hospitalized for major depression and was still an in-patient. She had not seen her little girl in several months, and prior to that time her care of the child had been limited. Mrs. A felt she lacked attachment to Betsy. She did not feel comfortable with her now that they were in each other's presence.

The first mother and child dyadic psychotherapy session was tense. Betsy cried when her nurse left the room. She at no time approached the therapist, though occasionally glancing in her direction. Betsy brought toys over to Mrs. A, who accepted them. Though Mrs. A reacted minimally to Betsy, she did not reach out to her. She was attentive and seemed pleased by the child's approach. Throughout the hour Betsy expressed no emotion of any kind, either in behavior or in facial expression. She was fearful of noises and maintained a hypervigilant attitude. Mrs. A was hurt in her recognition of Betsy's lack of attachment to her; Betsy did not care about leaving her mother. Throughout the next session Mrs. A continued to be highly anxious in her interactions with Betsy. She was able to state that she had been surprised at being pregnant (with Betsy), and then was fearful that Betsy would reject her. This was reflected in her manner of interactions. For example, her attempt to talk to her two-year-old was to ask her questions. Furthermore, the questions were worded negatively and fearfully: "You don't want to come with me?"

Therapy interventions were largely supportive. The emphasis was also on positive reinforcements by the therapist for nurturing behaviors on the mother's part and for reaching out on the child's part. Because there was so little of either of these behaviors forthcoming, guidance and behavioral directives were used. These interventions allowed for more, and more positive, warm interactions. After two dyadic psychotherapy sessions, Mrs. A was encouraged sufficiently in the improvements in her interactions with Betsy so that she twice visited the child at the orphanage between sessions. The change was dramatic in that Betsy was now sad when the mother left. By the start of the third session, Betsy no longer cried when the nurse left the room. Though the interactions had improved, Mrs. A was not making any physical contact with the child. The therapist modeled touching. Mrs. A's response was to use only her fingertips in touching Betsy. She said she felt funny with her. The therapist thought that though the child needed cuddling, this was a very difficult hurdle for the mother. In order to avoid too much delay in meeting this need of the child, strong intervention was indicated. The therapist therefore modeled playful physical interaction by taking Betsy's face in her hands, looking into her eyes, and playfully interacting. Betsy reacted with joy. Since the mother did not spontaneously initiate this, nor did she try it upon the therapist's suggestion, the therapist took the mother's hands, placed them on Betsy's face, and repeated the same interaction. With Betsy's joyful response to her, the mother was then able to move in the direction of physical contact with Betsy. Eye contact and playful holding were again encouraged in the fourth session. Mrs. A said that she had followed through on this when seeing Betsy at the orphanage, since the previous sessions.

Though the interactions were now more active, and Mrs. A was able to understand and act upon suggestions made by the therapist, she still felt a lack of relatedness to Betsy. The therapist suggested that Mrs. A interact with Betsy at the developmental level at which she had been when she had ceased taking care of her prior to her hospitalization. She was able to do so, for instance, changing Betsy's diaper (which she had not done during the previous contacts). This regression in their relationship seemed to function to allow Mrs. A to close the relatedness gap with her child. She consequently felt better. It seemed to repair a barrier between them.

During the following two weeks Mrs. A saw Betsy four times in the orphanage (missing a therapy session due to illness). In these visits she reported that she had been able to utilize the gains she had made during the previous sessions.

In the following, fifth, dyadic psychotherapy session, a drastic change was evidenced in Betsy's behavior and in the interactions with the mother. Betsy's anhedonia had lifted! She was bright-eyed, smiled, talked, and expressed joy. She was jumping up and down with joy at one point. She was much less constricted, exploring toys in the room, and actively and happily interacting, even so far as to make demands upon her mother. Mrs. A, in turn, was pleased. She put Betsy on her lap in order to be close to her. She kissed her and told her she loved her.

The institutional stare had been abandoned by this toddler. It had taken five dyadic psychotherapy sessions to accomplish this. The child lived in the orphanage during all of this time. The mother had been an in-patient during some of this time. She was now busy trying to arrange her life to work toward receiving her child back in her own care. The deeply pathological trend in the developmental process of this child had been rerouted. She was now on an essentially normal course of development.

Appendix D

Guide to Treatment Planning: A List of Standard Problems, Objectives, and Interventions

This guide is offered as an aide to therapists and to treatment teams. It offers the therapist a listing of frequent problems found so that he/she will be able to check this list for possible problem areas pertaining to the client. It is then possible to look at both standard objectives and interventions for these problems. This listing is not meant to be followed rigidly. There will be many other problem areas for any given client, and some of the listed problems may not apply. One can, however, use the listing to gain a general overview of problems found, related objectives, and interventions.

Treatment teams will also find the guide useful in their treatment planning, particularly where the problem-oriented method is used, for which this guide was written. It is divided into three broad areas: a list for expectant mothers, one for the infant, and another for the primary caretaker (mother), as the focus of the clinical intervention.

FOR EXPECTANT MOTHERS

Problem	Objective	Intervention
1. ambivalence about the pregnancy	decrease the ambivalence	exploration of conflict
2. improper physical care (drug abuse, lack of OB/GYN assessments, nutritional problems, hygiene, putting self at physical risk)	improve self-care	(a) pregnancy-oriented psychotherapy (b) counseling

Problem	Objective	Intervention
3. ambivalence about the disposition of the infant-to-be	resolution of conflicts	pregnancy-oriented psychotherapy
4. involving psychotic ideation in relation to the fetus/infant-to-be	dissolve the involving psychotic ideation	pregnancy-oriented psychotherapy
5. symptom formation due to self/or projected attribution in relation to pain of parturition	diminish the self/projected attribution	pregnancy-oriented psychotherapy

FOR THE INFANT

Problem	Objective	Intervention
1. markedly disturbed social relatedness	improve social relatedness	support mother's socializing interactions and infant's responses
2. persistent failure to intiate or respond to social interaction	improve infant's responsiveness toward others and spontaneity	support infant's spontaneous and responsive social interactions and mother's positive reactions to these
3. indiscriminate sociability	develop selective sociability	work on increasing positive attachment
4. floppiness (hypotonia)	normalize the muscle tone	physical therapy program integrated into a pleasurable mother/infant interaction within a social context
5. hypertonia (partial or generalized)	decrease the muscle tonus	sensory motor integration, program integrated into a pleasurable mother/infant interaction within a social context
6. lacking in ability to habituate	increased ability to habituate	psychoeducational with caretaker to protect the infant from overstimulation
7. fearfulness, markedly disturbed anxiety	reduce fear and anxiety	(a) assess source of fear (b) decrease the source of danger

Problem	Objective	Intervention
8. persistent gaze aversion	reversal of gaze aversion by development of eye contact	support the mother in this within dyadic psychotherapy
9. spinal arching when held by mother	reversal of spinal arching by development of molding	support mother's molding within dyadic psychotherapy
10. problems in consolability	increase consolability	help mother in her responsivity to child's needs
11. preference for inanimate objects (after 1 year of age)	increased emotional object relatedness	support the mother in increasing pleasurable interpersonal experiences
12. attention deficit	increased ability to focus attention	help the mother appropriately channel the child's attention
13. misconduct	decrease the misconduct	help the mother set appropriate limits
14. social withdrawal	lessen the withdrawal, increased sociability	increase object relatedness through dyadic psychotherapy
15. low energy and activity level, motor retardation	increase energy and activity level	work with mother to increase infant's stimulation
16. hyperactivity	decrease activity level	work with mother to soothe infant
17. disturbances in mood	stabilized mood	work with mother toward contingency in interactions
18. anhedonia	have the ability to experience pleasure	help the dyad to take pleasure in each other
19. irritability	decreased irritability	help the mother to provide a stable, comfortable environment
20. lack of evidence of directed behavior	develop goal-directed behavior	support the mother's use of rewards, and her phrasing of descriptions of behavior (to separate the goal from behavior aimed at achieving that goal)

Problem	*Objective*	*Intervention*
21. excessive compulsive absorption with tasks	reduce the excessive compulsive absorption with tasks	support family's positive interpersonal interactions with the child
22. lack of endurance	increased endurance	help the mother to provide patient presence and support to the child's endeavors

FOR THE PRIMARY CARETAKER (MOTHERS)

1. maternal attachment disorder	assessment of risk that there will be a separation	observations of mother/infant interactions
2. negative maternal attachment disorder	resolve the conflicts about separation	support the wish to separate
3. positive maternal attachment disorder	increase the positive maternal attachment	support the development of positive maternal attachment
4. feelings of anger at the child	decrease the anger	dyadic psychotherapy
5. impulsivity in expression of anger	decrease the impulsivity	(a) dyadic psychotherapy (b) focused therapy
6. persistent disregard for the child's emotional needs	develop caring behavior	heighten mother's consciousness for the child's needs and support attunement
7. disregard for the child's basic physical needs	mother to care for the child's physical needs	heighten mother's consciousness and knowledge of the child's physical needs
8. repeated change of primary caregiver	reduce the number of changes	advice to mothers, significant others, and/or child protective agencies
9. understimulation of infant	increase stimulating behavior	support mother's stimulating behavior
10. intrusive overstimulation of the infant	decrease intrusiveness	support mother's understanding of the infant's negative reaction to intrusiveness
11. non-contingent interactions with infant	increase contingency in interactions	support mother's emotional understanding of infant's communications

Appendix E

Typical Day Interview

This interview was developed by the author as an aide to under-standing the typical experiential conditions of the infant. It has been found extremely helpful, particularly when it is difficult to know the infant's situation between sessions. Through its use, it has been learned that the mother tends to be at her best during the sessions. It provides information concerning typical patterns of sleeping, eating, play, and contact with others, stimulation, and mood of the baby.

INSTRUCTIONS

The interviewer talks with the mother (the primary caretaker):

I would like to get an idea of what a typical day is like for _____ .

                                                                           (baby's name)

I would like you to pick one day last week that was typical (usual, regular, etc.) for _____ and you.
        (baby's name)

What day last week was typical? (when a day is chosen, ask her whether she was with her baby that day. Choose a day they were together.)

All right, now we are going to talk about that day (e.g., last Wednesday) only.

Think of last Wednesday.

What time did _____ wake up?

               (baby's name)

Where was _____ when he/she woke up?

           (baby's name)

In which room?

Who else was in the room?

What was _____ doing?

          (baby's name)

What sounds could _____ hear?

              (baby's name)

What mood was _____ in?

           (baby's name)

The interviewer helps the mother to answer as accurately as possible. *This is continued for each hour of the day (24 hrs.).* He/she then asks the mother questions so as to complete the second part of the form.

Note: The wording on the form is for the interviewer. He/she may change the wording to achieve maximum understanding by the mother.

Typical Day Interview

Name: Mother (interviewed) _____ Day chosen _____

Date of interview _____

Baby _____ Age _____ Birthdate _____

Time	Which Room	Where in room	Who else in Room	Activity	Sounds M-B Talking TV/Radio	Mood Baby Happy/ Crying
AM 7:						
8:						
9:						
10:						
11:						
PM 12:						
1:						
2:						
3:						
4:						
5:						
6:						
7:						
8:						
9:						
10:						
11:						
AM 12:						
1:						
2:						
3:						
4:						
5:						
6:						

Are any of the notations atypical for that day?_____

_____

Comments: _____

_____

_____

How do you put baby to sleep? _____

_____

Does he/she cry?_____

How long? _____

_____

Does baby understand "NO"? _____

_____

_____

What foods is baby eating?_____

Where does baby sit while eating? _____

Does baby eat by self? _____

   if not, who feeds him/her? _____

Are there visitors to the home?_____

   how many (who)? _____

_____

_____

Discipline: how? _____

         who does it? _____

         when? _____

   how are limits set for baby? _____

_____

Any comments? _____

_____

References

American Psychiatric Association. (1980). *Diagnostic and statistical manual of mental disorders* (3rd ed.). Washington, D.C.: American Psychiatric Association.

Beck, A. T. (1967). *Depression: Clinical, experimental, and theoretical aspects.* New York: Harper and Row.

Bender, L. (1956). Schizophrenia in childhood: Its recognition, description, and treatment. *American Journal of Orthopsychiatry, 26,* 499–506.

Bird, H. R. (1980). Stranger reaction vs. stranger anxiety. *Journal of the American Academy of Psychoanalysis, 8* (4), 555–563.

Brazelton, T. B. (1969). *Infants and mothers: Differences in development.* New York: Delacorte.

Brossard, M. (1974). The infant's conception of object permanence and the reaction to strangers. In T. G. Decarie (ed.), *The infant's reaction to strangers.* New York: International Universities Press.

Brossard, L. M., and Decarie, T. G. (1968). Comparative reinforcing effect of eight stimulations on the smiling response of infants. *Journal of Child Psychol, Psychiatry, 9,* 51–59.

Casler, L. (1965). The effect of supplementary verbal stimulation on a group of institutionalized infants. *Journal of Child Psychol, Psychiatry, 6,* 19–27.

Cicchetti, D. (1987). Developmental psychopathology in infancy: Illustration from the study of maltreated youngsters. *Journal of Consulting Psychology, 55,* 837–845.

Ferster, C. B., and Skinner, B. F. (1957). *Schedules of reinforcement.* New York: Appleton-Century-Crofts.

Fish, B. (1984). Characteristics and sequelae of the neurointegrative disorder in infants at risk for schizophrenia. In N. F. Watt, E. J. Anthony, L. C. Wynne, and J. E. Rolf (eds.), *Children at risk for schizophrenia* (pp. 423–439). Cambridge, Mass.: Cambridge University Press.

Fraiberg, S. (ed.). (1980). *Clinical studies in infant mental health.* New York: Basic Books.

Fraiberg, S. (1982). Pathological defenses in infancy. *Psychoanalytic Quarterly, 51* (4), 612–635.

Garmezy, N., and Phipps-Yonas, S. (1984). An early crossroad in research on risk for schizophrenia: The Dorado Beach Conference. In N. F. Watt, E. J. Anthony, L. C. Wynne, and J. E. Rolf (eds.), *Children at risk for schizophrenia* (pp. 6–18). Cambridge, Mass.: Cambridge University Press.

Garmezy, N., and Streitman, S. (1974, Spring). Children at risk: The search for the antecedents of schizophrenia: 1. Conceptual models and research models. *Schizophrenia Bulletin, 8,* 14–90.

Gochman, E. R. (1985). Bipolar mothering: Case description, mother-infant interactions and theoretical implications. *Child Psychiatry and Human Development, 16,* 120–125.

Gochman, E. R. (1986). Preventive therapy for high risk mothers and children. *Dynamic Psychotherapy, 4,* 34–39.

Gochman, E. R. (1988). Mother-infant dyadic psychotherapy. *Psychologist Psychoanalyst, 8* (3), 23.

Gochman, E. R. (1991). A conceptual statement on the attribution of worthlessness in depression. *Psychologist Psychoanalyst, 11* (2), 9.

Gochman, E.R.G. (1989a). A formulation of the psychodynamic purposiveness of a kidnapping: A brief report. *Psychoanalysis and Psychotherapy, 7* (1), 85–87.

Gochman, E.R.G. (1989b). A sense of panic in the infant. *Psychoanalysis and Psychotherapy, 7* (2), 162–165.

Gochman, E.R.G. (1992). A note on deep-seated social values and countertransference in mother-infant dyadic psychotherapy. *Psychoanalytic Psychology, 9* (3), 405–408.

Gochman, E. R., and Aisenstein, C. (1985). Exploration in high risk stimulation: Two modalities in mothering: *Eric Reports,* ED 249–715.

Greenspan, S. I. (1987). *Infants in multirisk families: Case studies in preventive intervention.* Madison, Conn.: International Universities Press.

Greenspan, S. I., and Lieberman, A. F. (1980). Infants, mothers and their interaction: A qualitative clinical approach to development assessment. *The course of life* (Vol. 1), Greenspan, S. I., and Pollock, G. H . (eds.). DHH Publication no. (ADM) 80–786.

Grubler, E. R. (1957). *Anxiety and perception: The relationship of two forms of anxiety to perception; A quantiative analysis of forces within the individual.* Ann Arbor, Mich.: University Microfilms.

Grunebaum, H., Weiss, J., Cohler, B. J., Hartman, C. R., and Gallant, D. H. (1975). *Mentally-ill mothers and their children.* Chicago: University of Chicago Press.

Haugan, G. M., and McIntire, R. W. (1972). Comparisons of vocal imitation, tactile stimulation, and food as reinforcers for infant vocalizations. *Developmental Psychology, 6,* 201–209.

Horner, A. (1980). The roots of anxiety, character structure, and psychoanalytic treatment. *Journal of the American Academy of Psychoanalysis, 8* (4), 565–573.

Korner, A. F. (1972). The relative efficacy of contact and vestibular proprioceptive stimulation in soothing neonates. *Child Development, 3* (1), 443–453.

Lennenberg, E. H. (1967). *Biological foundations of language.* New York: Wiley.

Murray, L., and Cooper, P. J. (1991). Postnatal depression and infant development. *British Medical Journal, 302,* 978–979.

Musick, J., Clark, R., Cohler, B., and Dincin, J. (1979, September). *Interactional patterns of schizophrenic, depressed and well mothers and their young children.* Paper presented at Annual Conference, American Psychological Association, New York.

Ornitz, E. M. (1970). Vestibular dysfunction in schizophrenia and childhood autism. *Community Psychiatry, 11,* 159–173.

Provence, S., and Lipton, R. C. (1962). *Infants in institutions.* New York: International Universities Press.

Sameroff, A. J. (1975, October). The children of mentally-disordered women: Neonatal characteristics. In *The Children of Schizophrenics.* Symposium conducted at the meeting of the American Academy of Child Psychiatry. Toronto, Ontario.

Schachter, J. (1970). Development of a screening questionnaire for schizophrenia. *Archives of General Psychiatry, 23,* 30–34.

Schachter, J., Kerr, J., Lachine, J. M., and Faer, M. (1975). Newborn offspring of a schizophrenic parent: Cardiac reactivity to auditory stimuli. *Psychophysiology, 12,* 483–492.

Schecter, D. (1980). Early developmental roots of anxiety. *Journal of the American Academy of Psychoanalysis, 8,* 538–554.

Seligman, M. (1975). *Helplessness: On depression, development and death.* San Francisco: Freeman.

Silverton, L., Finello, K., and Mednick, S. (1983). Children of schizophrenic women: Early factors predictive of schizophrenia. *Infant Mental Health Journal, 4,* 202–215.

Slucking, W. (1964). *Imprinting and early learning.* London: Mentheren.

Sobel, D. E. (1961). Children of schizophrenic patients: Preliminary observations on early development. *American Journal of Psychiatry, 118,* 512.

Spielberger, C. D. (ed.). (1972). *Anxiety: Current trends in theory and research.* New York: Academic Press.

Spitz, R., in collaboration with Cobliner, G. (1965). *The first year of life.* New York: International Universities Press.

Stevens, B. C. (1971). Psychoses associated with childbirth: A demographic survey since the development of community care. *Social Science Medicine, 5,* 527–543.

Watt, N. F., Anthony, E. J., Wynne, L. C., and Rolf, J. E. (eds.). (1984). *Children at risk for schizophrenia: A longitudinal perspective.* Cambridge, Mass.: Cambridge University Press.

Weary, G., and Mirel, H. L. (1982). *Integration of clinical and social psychology.* New York: Oxford University Press.

Werner, E. E. (1989). *Vulnerable, but invincible: A longitudinal study of resilient children and youth.* New York: Adams, Bannister, Cox.

Wright, E. L. (1971, April). A correlational study of selected sociological variables and two ranges of Stanford-Binet Intelligence quotients among culturally disadvantaged preschool children. *Dissertation Abstracts International, 31* (10-A), 5219.

Wynne, L. C. (1984). The University of Rochester Child and Family Study: Overview of research plan. In N. F. Watt, E. J. Anthony, L. C. Wynne, and J. E. Rolf (eds.),

Children at risk for schizophrenia (pp. 335–347). Cambridge, Mass.: Cambridge University Press.

Yarrow, L. J. (1961). Maternal deprivation: Toward an empirical and conceptual re-evaluation. *Psychological Bulletin, 58,* 459–490.

Yarrow, L. J., Rubenstein, J. L., and Pedersen F. (1975). *Infant and environment: Early cognitive and motivational development.* Washington, D.C.: Hemisphere Publishing Corp.

Index

About the Author

EVA R. GRUBLER GOCHMAN is Director of the Parent and Infant Development Program, Commission on Mental Health Services, Department of Human Services, District of Columbia. The program began under the auspices of the National Institute of Mental Health at St. Elizabeth's Hospital. She also does Superior Court ordered forensic psychological assessments of abused and neglected children and their families. Her private practice is in Potomac, Maryland. She is a Diplomate in Clinical Psychology (American Board of Professional Psychology), and is a fellow of the Academy of Clinical Psychology. Gochman has lived and taught in Europe and Puerto Rico. She has coauthored (with S. I. Gochman) *A Psychological Profile of the Puerto Rican University Student* (1976).

ISBN 0-275-94927-3

EAN

9 780275 949273

HARDCOVER BAR CODE